FIGHTING
WITH CRIB GLOVES

RICHARD KEANE

FIGHTING
WITH CRIB GLOVES

My Battle with Cystic Fibrosis

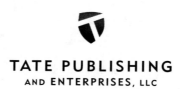

TATE PUBLISHING
AND **ENTERPRISES**, LLC

Published by Tate Publishing & Enterprises, LLC
127 E. Trade Center Terrace | Mustang, Oklahoma 73064 USA
1.888.361.9473 | www.tatepublishing.com

Tate Publishing is committed to excellence in the publishing industry. The company reflects the philosophy established by the founders, based on Psalm 68:11,
"The Lord gave the word and great was the company of those who published it."

Book design copyright © 2014 by Tate Publishing, LLC. All rights reserved.
Cover design by Anne Gatillo
Interior design by Gram Telen

Published in the United States of America

ISBN: 978-1-63063-153-6
1. Biography & Autobiography / Medical
2. Medical / General
14.01.10

To Valerie, my sweet sister, my friend, and my hero, who, in 1976 at age eighteen, succumbed to pneumonia and tuberculosis as a result of cystic fibrosis. Although she suffered terribly for a number of years, Val fought hard, never quit and refused to indulge in self-pity. The last thing she told me was to keep fighting…I haven't stopped.

My sisters—Mary Lou, Amy, Julie, Jennifer—and my brothers—Scott, Timmy, and Gregg—have each in their own way, not only helped mold me into the person I am today, but also inspired me to write these memoirs and to live.

Dr. Jack Gorvoy, my dear friend, after taking care of me for forty-five years, gave me something for which I can never repay…time.

For my father, who I am doing my best to forgive…I miss you.

My mother, the most decent, caring, and nurturing person I will ever know, has in no small way, made me the person I am today. I have no words to express the love and gratitude I have for my mother.

MaryAnne, my wife and friend, you are the sole reason I am still here. There are so many things to thank you for, so I'll keep it simple; thank you for saving my life.

Each of the fore mentioned have impacted my life in ways none of them will ever truly understand. To say I feel privileged and fortunate to have lived long enough to let them each know this, is an understatement.

Contents

Introduction

For those of us born with a life-threatening disease, such as cystic fibrosis (CF), emotional support from family and friends can never be overstated. So much so, that in the case of CF patients who are seeking lung transplants, strong family support, emotional, and physical are part of the criteria required before some institutions will consider one an eligible transplant candidate.

I have been very fortunate in this regard as my very large family, my wife and our best friends, Susan and Peter have always been there for me with unconditional love and support.

I believe it important for those reading these memoirs to know a little something about each of my brothers and sisters so that the diversity in personalities and the love that made growing up in a large family inspiring to me is understood.

When my older sister, Mary Lou and I were young children, we had our share of arguments and fights as brothers and sisters do. I was raised not to hit girls, so if it did get physical, I was always on the losing end. When we were young, Mary Lou found a particularly sensitive spot on my back just below my shoulder blade and then proceeded to pound that spot for the next ten years. I swear to her now that I still get stiffness there once in a while. Of course I don't, but it worked (until now) in making her feel guilty.

As adults now, I feel and I hope she does also as close as any brother can be to his older sister. We talk, play a little golf, and laugh a little almost every time we get together, usually with me, and sometimes at me. I don't care which as long as she is happy.

She has been a godsend and best friend to our mother, whom she has kept company and lived with for many years. As the older sister continues to look after her younger brother, Mary Lou has given of her time in many ways. Her assistance with the writing, construction, and completion of my book will forever be appreciated. Thank you, Lulu.

Amy was given the name Happy by our father, who was being extremely sarcastic at the time. To say, she is a little over emotional doesn't really cut it. She is also the owner of a huge heart and will do anything and everything she can to help anyone in need. Amy has had her own serious health issues to deal with during her life, including an aneurism found lodged deep in her brain in 2008. It remains, unfortunately, an ongoing problem for Amy. Depression episodes have come and gone throughout her life and surely this latest problem with the aneurism hasn't improved the situation. Surgeries have been performed to try and alleviate the headaches, seizures, and other symptoms she is suffering as a result. The perseverance Amy displays to remain *happy* and the smile she wears despite these issues, has kept her outlook positive.

My beautiful sister Julie has also had her own difficulties with health as she underwent open heart surgery at age six. While undergoing a sweat test checking for CF, it was discovered that the left ventricle of her tiny heart was clogged. Ironically, had I and Valerie not had CF, Julie's condition may not have been detected and would have been life-threatening. See, I was good for something while I was a child, Mom. The surgery, however, could not be performed until her body had developed further and was strong enough to withstand such a procedure.

Having gotten *that* out of the way, allow me now to tell you that we are pretty sure Julie is from another planet. We are not completely sure which planet, and perhaps, it has not yet been discovered. Wherever it is, I believe to survive there, one must work each day until they actually collapse or risk being shunned by society.

Julie graduated from Molloy College top of her class way back when and is obviously very bright. She has always been my greatest fan and laughs at just about all my comedic comments and antics.

Julie met her husband, Tom, about thirty years ago, shortly after he had suffered a terrible accident. At the young age of nineteen, Tom was left paralyzed from the waist down. I can remember asking myself, when I found out they had become engaged, if Julie was really going to be able to handle the reality of living with someone whose physical capabilities will forever be limited. It never became even close to an issue for her, and the love she and Tom have for and show toward each other transcends any obstacles they may encounter. Julie is that special kind of person. True love. Priceless.

I've always found it interesting that as good a cook as my mother was, none of her daughters came close to matching her prowess in the kitchen. Relax girls, I know some of you cook a little, but you're not quite up there with Mom. Three out of the four boys, however, are in the food service business.

Scott, though, is the leader of the pack. An executive chef in an exclusive country club in Boca Raton, Florida, Scott's culinary talent and hard work has earned him a much respected name amongst the sunshine state's top country clubs. While a senior in Baldwin High School, Scott won a countywide cooking contest and earned a trip to the renowned Concord Hotel in upstate New York to participate in a state wide contest. Scott then attended the Culinary Institute in New York and proceeded after graduation to pursue his dream.

He is an amazing father to his three children. Scott, by the way, is not vain like his older brother, and that's a good thing as he won the title of best-looking as a senior in high school. Now if I had won, I would have printed a tee shirt with my picture on the back and would still be wearing it today, tattered as it might be by now. Just kidding...there would also certainly be a picture of me on the front.

A naturally gifted athlete since childhood, Timmy provided thrills for me as I watched him play sports at such a high-level and at such a young age. I envied the relative ease with which he displayed his strength and athleticism. I played those same sports at a decent talent level, but I will admit I was very jealous watching him. There were times when I was angry that I was born with such a thin physique because of CF and was always envious of his. I guess you have to make the best of what you're born with, and I *did* get the good hair

My three brothers were bunched together in age, and though I was a good number of years older than them, I would get some little games of football going when they were kids, and we would have a blast. I've always wondered what my life would have been like if I had grown up with a brother around my age, but alas, nothing but women. Timmy has a fantastic football mind and has coached at a number of different age levels. I'm still hoping the New York Jets give him a call; they could use him. Tim has a wonderful family and like all my siblings with children—caring, loving, and involved parents with their kids. Tim's only daughter, Jessica, is one of four god children I am proud to call mine.

Gregg, my youngest brother, for some crazy reason thinks he is as quick-witted as or funnier than I am.... very disturbing. He and his family live in Long Beach, California, and he doesn't miss a chance to let me know how perpetually beautiful the weather is out there. Gregg owns a catering business, and again, as all my siblings are, he is a very hard worker. As busy as Gregg is with his business, he remains very involved with his two boys' sports activities and their schooling. Gregg is also the only family member I have that could give me a run for my money when it comes to self-vanity. All right, I admit it...he has the dark tan, movie star looks, and has always been better looking than me but *not* funnier, sorry buddy.

My beautiful sister and goddaughter Jenny, is the youngest in the family at forty -four years of age. She has earned two degrees during the course of her life and is now a professional photographer. She has accomplished all of this while battling cystic fibrosis. Thankfully, aside from a few hospital admissions during her childhood and teen years, Jen did not experience too difficult a time with CF until her mid-thirties.

When she was a child, I would pray she wouldn't go through what Valerie did, and this particular prayer did get answered for me…and her. I grew up around CF children and CF adults and have seen too many of them suffer harshly with the disease.

A good many people with CF have a certain *look* to them regarding clubbed fingertips and slightly hunched backs as I will explain to you as you read on. Jennifer, though, is an anomaly. She was an adorable little girl who grew into a gorgeous young woman and easily could have modeled for a living. To be honest, when I was younger, I kept waiting for her body to start to deteriorate as CF worked its evil magic, but thankfully, that never happened. She has always been active with skiing, bike riding, and working out, and I am certain this has helped in keeping her strong well into her forties.

The college degree she earned in nursing, allowing her to work at Long Island Jewish Medical Center for over ten years in the pediatric ICU and post-op units, was not only beneficial to her, but to me as well. Any questions I've had over the years regarding many of my health issues, I've had only to pick up the phone and ask Jenny. Most times, Jen was able to answer these questions. If not, she often would know where to get those answers. She helped me tremendously in the months before my transplant, allowing me to talk about my issues for long stretches of time while she kept my attitude positive and my demeanor calm. The same held true after transplant as she kept me comforted and reassured about all I was experiencing.

I believe, as difficult as this disabling disease Jenny and I share can be, the fact that we share it and can relate to each other on that level has made the journey we both are going through, a little more bearable. Oh, and by the way, Jenny and her daughter, Dara who is also my goddaughter are VIP members of the Richie Keane fan club.

My life, physically, has not been easy, but having been blessed with the family I've been blessed with has kept me emotionally upbeat and driven. I will be forever thankful for them.

Having often been in a hospital setting throughout my life, I have seen many people—young and old—suffer from illnesses that surely test their emotional and physical reserve. Cystic fibrosis is just one of these illnesses, and I have had a ringside seat to witness this disease's consequences.

As a child with CF, I would sit in clinic, really not understanding why I was coughing so much, and what my body was going through. However, witnessing the desperate physical condition some of the children in that same clinic were in, even at my young age, I understood this was a serious deal.

I don't know why I was born with this incurable genetic disease. I have stopped asking myself that question. As I've grown older and seen how much suffering—in all manner—other people have had to deal with, I am humbled and quieted. Well, quieted occasionally anyway.

I only know that the chromosomes responsible for my brown hair, my brown eyes, and my astonishingly quick wit were also responsible for my battle with cystic fibrosis.

Preface

There have been a number of books written on the subject of cystic fibrosis, some factual and statistical, others, personal hardships and triumphs. My story touches on each of these, hopefully with some humor sprinkled in. I write about my life at this time because in one month, at age fifty-five, I will have reached the five year anniversary of my double lung transplant. Not only will this book bring more exposure to the CF plight but hopefully will also bring to light an understanding that despite whatever difficulties one goes through in his or hers life, no matter how extreme they may be, laughter, optimism, and personal goals must always be your priorities.

Some of the many health issues mentioned in the book are difficult for me to write about, but good times and bad will be revealed here. This is, after all, a story of faith and perseverance. Faith in God and one's self, and the perseverance to live and to fight any obstacles that might keep you from the life and people you love.

For those who do not know what CF is, here is a basic history and definition. The facts and statistics I site throughout the book have been acquired from the internet site, CysticFibrosis.com.

The symptoms of what was most likely cystic fibrosis were first documented in the mid-1800s. There is literature from the 1700s that describe symptoms of an illness at that time that some scientists believe could very well have been CF. Although CF is considered a rare disease, it is the most common, deadly, inherited disease affecting Caucasians in the United States. The CF gene was discovered in 1938 by *Dr. Dorothy Andersen, a pathologist at New York's Babies Hospital.* In 1985, scientists identified chromosome 7 as the culprit causing the defective genes responsible for CF. Interestingly, though known now primarily as a lung disease, it was originally named *cystic fibrosis of the pancreas.*

There are now approximately 30,000 children and adults afflicted with CF in the United States and 70,000 worldwide. One in every 4,000 children are born with CF. One in every 29 Caucasians are born with the CF gene. For a person to be born with CF, the abnormal, mutated gene must be present in both parents. Though the disease has been diagnosed throughout the world, it originated in northern Europe. Ireland has the highest number of people affected per capita, but most people with CF live here in the United States.

In 1955, one year before I was born, the Cystic Fibrosis Foundation was formed to encourage and fund research. At that time, the majority of CF patients did not reach even one or two years of age.

CF is a chronic, progressive, hereditary disease that attacks primarily the respiratory and digestive systems. The reproductive, immune, and circulatory systems are also adversely affected. An over-secretion of mucus in the lungs clogs the bronchial tubes and airways, and because it is so thick, it becomes very difficult to cough up and get rid of. This buildup of mucus finds places in the lungs and airways to sit and fester so as to allow infection and consequently pneumonia to occur. A scar is left in the lung at the site of each infection. Multiple pneumonias eventually leave the lungs so damaged and scarred that lung capacity is diminished to the point where oxygen is needed and inevitably transplant if one is eligible for such a procedure.

There is no cure for cystic fibrosis. The average life expectancy now, in 2012, for one stricken with CF is thirty-six years. There has been progress toward new treatments and medicines, but it will still take years of testing, trials for genetic therapies, and USDA approval for new antibiotics before they can go from concepts and theories to cure.

For now, personal goals, achievements, laughter, and love of life are my motivations. I am not and will not be defined by cystic fibrosis. The love I have for my wife, my family, music, sports, and laughter is who I am. I am a fighter of a terminal, chronic illness that takes courage, patience, and faith in my physical and mental strength to defeat. I am a CF victor...not a victim. There is a life, however long it may be, that must be lived. And...there is hope.

Crib Gloves

Dr. Sheldon Miller hung the little black boxing gloves on the corner of the crib, looked at the young woman—my mother—and told her it would be a tough road but that her son is a fighter. I will need to wear those gloves everyday for the rest of my life. I can loosen them from time to time, but I can never take them off.

Not much at all was known about cystic fibrosis in 1956, the year I was born in South Nassau Hospital in Oceanside New York. Most children didn't live long enough for doctors to be able to gather any conclusive findings, and of course, they had to let my mother know this. A very difficult thing to hear as a young parent, I would imagine.

Only a handful of doctors around the world had even heard of the disease let alone study and research it. As with any *healthy* newborn, I was able to go home with my mother just a few days after being welcomed to the world. I weighed in at seven pounds, five ounces and looked like most newborns, though probably a bit cuter than most. However, only a week or so passed before symptoms of CF first became evident. I was not digesting properly and therefore, not receiving the proper nutrition required for an infant. I began to lose weight rapidly. Breastfeeding was discontinued by the doctor and various baby formulas were introduced but with no success. This loss of weight and malnutrition continued for about ten weeks, resulting in an admission to Nassau County Medical Center. Dr. Miller, the pediatrician assigned me, after observing me as an infant, battle measles and chicken pox along with other complications, all within weeks of each other, instructed that I be quarantined until further studies could be made. I remained in quarantine for seven months. One night during those months, as my mother was entering the hospital to come see me, she was met by Dr. Miller and was informed that I had stopped breathing for a short time earlier that afternoon, but was revived quickly and was stable. The doctor then told my mother he had an idea of what might be the cause of these problems.

While a young pediatrician doing his residency at Meadowbrook Hospital on Long Island in New York, he had kept up to date, as much as one could without the internet, on all known and newly discovered pediatric diseases, disorders, and treatments. After further testing and research, Dr. Miller then diagnosed me with the rare disease, cystic fibrosis. Most babies born with CF were usually not surviving for more than a year or so, with many infants dying soon after birth. My mother was prepared to lose her child to this disease. At the very least, she would now be able to put a name to the illness her son had and begin to learn about and better deal with it.

I can't imagine how harrowing those first two years of rocking to sleep or should I say, trying to rock to sleep a sick child must have been. To make matters even more frustrating for Mom, many times after I would finally get to sleep, it would be time for my physical therapy. This is when she would have to pound my chest and back to help loosen the mucus filling my tiny lungs. Of course, this would upset me to no end. She tells me how after she would try for hours to stop me from crying, of course to no avail, she would join me in a duet of blood curdling cries and screams. How adorable was I? Of course, later, she realized the constant crying was due to my continuous hunger pains.

I have tried to track Dr. Miller down and will continue to do so. I would love to thank him personally for his caring, his faith in me, and the boxing gloves.

Thank you, Dr. Miller, for helping me win the first of many rounds in this lifelong fight.

Dr. Jack Gorvoy

With so little known about my disease at this point and with a weak immune system allowing all these problems, I was transferred to the only hospital on Long Island treating children with CF—Long Island Jewish Hillside Medical Center (LIJHMC) of New Hyde Park on Long Island.

In 1949, LIJHMC opened a clinic run by Dr. Jack Gorvoy, a pediatrician from Toronto, who was making the study and treatment of CF his life's work. While aiding me in the research of my book, Dr. Gorvoy told me he first became interested in the disease when he was a young doctor doing his residency at Bellevue Hospital in New York.

One year, a young couple who lived down the block from Dr. Gorvoy had a new baby boy who was having trouble digesting and unable to gain weight. Aware that their neighbor, Dr. Gorvoy, was a pediatrician, the couple asked him to accept their child as one of his patients. Other doctors had examined and tested the child but were coming to no conclusions as to why he was continuing to lose weight and not responding to medications. Dr. Gorvoy, after running some of his own tests and making his own observations, had suspicions these symptoms were a result of cystic fibrosis, a fairly recently discovered children's disease. It perplexed the young doctor as to why so little could be done for the baby so much so that he became immersed in the research and study of cystic fibrosis.

When Dr. Gorvoy finally gave the okay to discharge me after about two years of intermittent hospitalizations, my mother brought home a beautiful, bouncing, adorable two-year-old boy. I believe it was about a week later when my mother called the hospital to see if there was anything else they wanted to test me for...and to please take their time in doing so.

So began my fifty-five-year relationship with the most giving, caring, and brilliant person I will ever know. Now ninety-four, Dr. Gorvoy is known worldwide for his work with cystic fibrosis and has been published many times over. His tireless effort, selflessness, and dedication are the main reasons the life expectancy of CF patients has gone from only a few months to thirty-six years in my lifetime.

Sweatin' it Out

In the sixties, my formidable years, if you were to watch me in action for more than let's say, a minute, you would have described me as "a very active child." You would have been being very polite. Looking back, I'm sure I had a good, healthy case of Attention Deficit Disorder (ADD) with a touch of Obsessive Compulsive Disorder (OCD) thrown in. Just in case there were any doubts about my *professional* diagnosis, my father had taken a video camera and filmed me in action when I was about ten years old, most likely for future evidence.

Apparently, one beautiful spring day, my parents thought it might be fun to take a few of the kids with some friends down to Silver Lake, our neighborhood pond. In the video, the gang is seen sitting on a park bench, readying themselves for pictures. There is a hold up, though. One child is circling the bench at high speed, and for no apparent reason. I'm fairly sure, looking back now, my parents probably wanted to strangle me at times. I'm also assuming, no, I'm hoping that deep down, they were happy to see so much energy from a son they almost lost as an infant to illness. Perhaps they were not feeling grateful at that specific moment though. What a pain in the ass I must have been.

One summer, I recall a family trip to Carson City, a western theme park in upstate New York. After arriving and unloading the bunch of us, Dad gathered us up and gave us our instructions on behavior for the day. As we started toward the entrance, I felt a sharp pain in my buttocks. Dad had kicked me in the ass, hard. I asked him why, knowing I had done nothing wrong, yet. He responded by saying he knew that at some point during the day, I would annoy him, and he didn't want other people to see him give me a boot. As it turned out, this was basically a preemptive strike. Such a thoughtful man he was. I will add this though, any time I did get hit or punished, and it wasn't often, I'm sure I deserved it.

When I see what's going on in the world these days, I realize how fortunate I was to grow up when and where I did. We had a great neighborhood with quite a few children. Without the aid of iPads and computers, believe it or not, we actually had fun *physically* playing together, imagine that.

The only real CF issue I can recall interfering with my childhood years were frequent visits to the hospital for checkups and a lot of what my best friend Steve Funk called *shriveling up*.

With extreme exertion, and that was common for me, intense coughing fits would follow. With the heavy build up of mucus, breathing became very difficult during these episodes. The *shriveling up*, as it were, was the hunching of my shoulders inward while coughing to try and alleviate the discomfort that came with these coughing episodes. This hunching action also expanded the lungs to maximize air intake.

Any vigorous activity I take part in, especially in hot weather, causes me to sweat profusely. So much so that the amount of salt lost from my body actually becomes visible as it dries and crystallizes on the skin of my arms and legs. It's actually very cool to look at if one can describe it as such. It's the little things that get me excited, you see. When one loses this much salt from the body, strength and energy is acutely depleted.

While pitching in a baseball game as a nine-year-old Little Leaguer, I lost so much salt through my sweat pores and became so exhausted from the extreme heat we were playing in that I collapsed. The same scenario occurred eight years later while in high school during a football practice. Even with the salt pills we were given by the coach at that time, the vast amount of salt and strength lost while sweating so profusely is hard for anyone's body to overcome, especially mine.

This is why the first test done to determine if a person has CF is the sweat test. This test is basically the gold standard when it comes to diagnosing CF in any infant, child, or adult. The amount or level of chloride (salt) contained in the CF person is considerably higher than that of a person without the disease. If that level number meets the criteria set for CF, that individual most likely has the disease. This is not the absolute, confirmed diagnosis of the disease as further testing is required, but the overwhelming chances are that CF is present.

Being actively involved in sports was always a big part of my childhood and continues to be now. Remember, in the sixties, not only were there no Xboxes, Atari's first video game, Pong, wasn't even invented yet!

As kids, we were always outside running around like banshees, having to be called in just about every night. I may have been the lone banshee, and the others might have been just running around like normal children, now that I reflect further on it. I realized, though, a long time ago that I should be thankful for the high energy I was born with. I truly believe if I hadn't been hyper, and occasionally annoying, I wouldn't be writing this book now.

Heart and Soul

As often and as hard as I pushed my sister Valerie to "get in the game," she very rarely did. She was a little timid when it came to taking part in our children's games that required physical exertion. Born in 1958, Val was two years younger than me. She was given a sweat test soon after birth and tested positive for CF. Due to my own array of health issues triggered by CF, Valerie was immediately started on a regimen of antibiotics and physical therapy to keep her lungs clear. She was slight as a child and remained so through adolescence. Doctors and nutritionists put her on special diets to encourage a weight gain, but with no real success. Though Val did have some relatively mild issues with her lungs as a child, it wasn't until she reached her young teens that serious infections began to occur. Fortunately for my mother, she didn't have to watch her second child in a row suffer terribly as an infant or as a young child from the wrath of cystic fibrosis.

From time to time, Val would decide she had the energy to take part in our games and activities, and her reward for that decision would be the inevitable coughing fit that followed. This was difficult and discouraging for her, to say the least.

Our neighbors knew very little if anything about our disease as did we, but we all *heard* the symptoms of it. The coughing that Val and I couldn't avoid, even as children, was unfortunately attention getting and difficult to listen to. Our neighbors became so concerned with this harsh, deeply congestive cough Valerie was exhibiting; they became understandably concerned as to whether their children could catch anything from her, or me, for that matter.

Our neighbors called a meeting amongst themselves and discussed their concerns on the issue. Valerie was loved by all in the neighborhood, but this was an issue they believed had to be addressed. One of the women called on my mother and discussed the situation. My mother explained that their children are not at any risk as a result of her coughing. The irony of this situation is that their children's occasional colds and viruses posed much more of a risk to Valerie's health than did she to theirs. The matter was dropped.

Valerie was a very pretty girl whose dark hair and complexion prompted me to tease her about perhaps being adopted. So this thin little girl, who often refused to play any games that would certainly exhaust her, decided at ten years of age to take horseback riding lessons. A nice game of tag made Val a little nervous, but she showed no fear as she mounted a 1,200-pound animal. You have to admire that. Her bravery far surpassed what mine could ever be, and it served her well throughout her short life. There aren't many people in the world who were more gentle and peaceful than her. Even when cystic fibrosis began, seemingly with a purpose, to work its disruptive and destructive self into her life, her selflessness and bravery never wavered.

I had already experienced multiple pneumonias by the time Valerie's lungs started their rapid decline. I knew all too well what suffering was in store for my closest sibling. Closest, not only in age, but in friendship and the commonality we shared growing up and battling this disease.

I have so many memories of Valerie that I couldn't possibly recall them all and wouldn't want to do so as some of them are too emotional for me to delve into. As young children, we did everything together, such as watching scary movies from behind the recliners in the den to putting on (Broadway worthy) Christmas plays with my older sister Mary Lou. Some of my fondest memories though, are the times we danced together. I have a photo of her and me, ballroom dancing, and yes, we're going to call it that, at ages nine and seven. We always loved to dance and sing. My absolute favorite memories of Valerie and me, were of the many times we played "Heart and Soul" on our piano together as children and then as teens.

Music was always a big part of mine and Valerie's lives, whether singing Christmas carols with our family, or just listening to my "forty-fives" as a teenager. Certainly not a claim to fame, but I sang the song "Edelweiss" from the movie, *The Sound of Music*, in a duet with a classmate in the second grade. We rocked the auditorium. Every Christmas, when all my aunts, uncles, cousins, and family would gather round to sing Christmas Carols, I would be urged to sing my solo rendition of "Edelweiss." I did not need much urging to do so. Where was *American Idol* when I needed it?

As teens in concert choir throughout our years in high school, my buddy Steve and I had to put up with some serious ribbing from our friends about our exquisite singing voices. Are we noting sarcasm? Now though, I am relegated to only dancing.

If Valerie were here today, I know she would agree with me in saying we had a happy and harmonious childhood.

A Price to Pay

Valerie and I remained very close as we entered our teens, and my friends, although a couple of years older than hers, became and remained friends for years to come. I'll always remember and admire Donna, Rosemary, Carol, Mary Chris, and Doreen for the special love and respect each showed toward Valerie. They were her closest friends and were there for her until the end. They were always in awe of her dignity, strength, and reserve while they watched, sadly and helplessly, as her health and body deteriorated over the last few years of her life.

As her body was weakened even further by CF, I got angrier and angrier at God for allowing this. I would pray every night for her infections and suffering to somehow be transferred to me. A very naïve and desperate prayer, indeed, but I knew I could handle any infections given me, and I knew she could not. I genuinely and honestly thought my prayers would help. I still say the same prayers regarding my sister Jenny, with so far, better results. At least I believe my prayers have helped.

The nights I lay in bed with the pillow wrapped around my head to mute Val's horrific choking and coughing fits were countless. I truly remember those nights as if they had just passed. It's very difficult for me to recall and describe to you the horrible gurgling and choking sounds that seemed to and sometimes did go on for hours and hours. Often, I would go into her room and try to console and calm her while she was trying to rid herself of this vile mucus. The more she cried, the more she coughed. Any exertion at all, whether crying, laughing or just about anything else that required physical energy, would trigger a coughing fit. CF wouldn't let her go.

Coughing and gasping for breath for hours on end is a common occurrence for the CF person with an active lung infection. When you finally feel like you have gotten everything cleared out of your lungs and are able to calm your breathing down, another full on attack ensues all too often and too quickly. I have always been astounded and angered at how quickly the CF lungs produce this mucus. Until my transplant, this was the most frustrating aspect of the disease for me, not the lack of breath in my lungs and not the multitude of infections but the constant, rapid accumulation of mucus.

It was explained to me by one doctor that one reason the mucus accumulated so rapidly was due to the tiny, fine hairs called cilia we all have, lining the bronchial tubes in the lungs. In normal lungs, the cilium flow in one direction, allowing mucus—which we all have in our lungs—to move along smoothly. In CF patients, the cilium flow in erratic, random directions and bunches up the mucus. The CF person also lacks an enzyme that helps to thin out the mucus, and this is also a major factor. With the mucus being thinner, it becomes much easier to expectorate, or spit up.

I've always known, that as repulsive as it was, I had to do my best to cough as hard as I could and get the mucus out of my lungs and airways. This is a very difficult and exhausting process that requires every bit of strength you can muster. All the muscles in the back, abdomen, and chest must be used to achieve this.

This is truly a revolting process that Valerie could not or would not do enough of. I would implore her to cough it out but had little success. I would sit with Valerie on the edge of her bed during these episodes until she caught her breath, and after saying the usual, "You'll be okay" and "Don't cry, Val," I would put my hand on her leg, look at her, and smile. I could always draw a smile out of her no matter how terrible she was feeling.

This gift of mine to make people laugh was and always has been my strongest suit. After all, I *was* voted wittiest as a senior in high school. Often, though, making Valerie laugh would trigger a wave of guilt over me. After exerting the energy to laugh, there was always a price to pay for my sister. I did love to make her laugh though because to see this quiet, subdued little girl just lose it and crack up laughing was a satisfying victory for me.

Val's End Stage

As her hospitalizations became more frequent and for longer durations, Valerie's spirit bent a little, but never broke. I can't begin to tell you about the number of tests she and I have undergone, just to say it was for her and remains so for me—never ending.

The only test or procedure my sister was afraid of was an arterial blood gas, or ABG as the doctors put it. This test is performed by the technician sticking a needle at a ninety degree angle directly into the wrist at the site of one's pulse or artery. I recall her anger at the fact that in her last weeks of life, they were still performing this extremely painful test on her. I understand the doctors were trying to learn, but Valerie was basically a guinea pig at that juncture of her life. This is a tough reality for me to get my head around, but many CF patients, like Valerie and myself had to suffer these painful procedures to help the CF patients of the future live longer. These kids and young adults who endured these procedures are true heroes.

During one of the last visits I had with Val, she told me not to let them give me a blood gas, unless Dr. Gorvoy thought it was necessary. There is a numbing agent now injected at the site where blood will be drawn, but I am still afraid of this test and no other.

There were a number of times we were both hospitalized at the same time; two or three of those times during the last couple of years of her life. She was in bed most of the time, so I would go down to visit her and try to push her to take a walk with me, but mostly I visited her to cheer her up and to make her smile.

It was difficult to watch Valerie as she approached end stage cystic fibrosis. It was especially difficult for my mother to watch. I can't know what watching your child suffer, the way my sister did, can do to a parent. As for my father, he very rarely visited Valerie or me while we were in the hospital. I know he loved us but was not ever able to emotionally handle the consequences of having children with CF.

As I watched my mother travel back and forth to the hospital everyday and night during those years, I made the decision to only allow my mother to come once in a while to see me during my hospitalizations. Personally, although I appreciated their concern, I never was comfortable with visitors, family or otherwise, while I was sick.

Missing quite a bit of her last two years of high school due to numerous hospitalizations, Valerie insisted on keeping up with her classmates academically. She loved school, was very bright, and insisted her homework be brought to her at the hospital. Valerie was so well-liked by students and faculty alike that the principal of Baldwin Senior High School arranged a bedside graduation ceremony at Long Island Jewish

Hospital at the end of the school year. I know Valerie could not have been more proud or more thankful for this thoughtful gesture.

Soon after her graduation, Valerie was diagnosed with tuberculosis. *Thank God because I believe she was beginning to get bored with only frequent pneumonia infections.* I know some people say that God gives people only what they can handle, but this just seemed cruel to me.

At some point in early December of 1976, Valerie wrote in her diary that she knew her time here was short but wanted to live through one more Christmas with her family.

Valerie died December 23, 1976. It was the first Christmas our mother didn't have the whole family and our relatives over to our house. We buried my sister two days after Christmas. Cystic Fibrosis doesn't let go. My God, do I miss my sister.

Climbing the Rose

An increase in the identification and diagnosis of CF in young children and infants was evident in 1955. Not a common hereditary disease at the time—only 1 in 4000 people diagnosed—this increase spawned the Cystic Fibrosis Foundation that year.

In 1965, Richard Weiss, a four-year-old boy with CF, overheard his mother on the phone talking about him and thought he heard her say that he had "sixty-five roses." She passed that story on to the Palm Beach, Florida, chapter of the foundation, and they adopted the name for their annual CF fund raiser ball. Sixty-five roses still is recognized in many countries as an extension of the CF foundation. You can't make this stuff up. Unwittingly, of course, the boy heard what actually is a perfect metaphor for the disease.

A rose, the ancient symbol for love, is a beautiful flower with a unique scent but also has sharp thorns that can cause pain. Suffering the thorn sticks of cystic fibrosis is not only painful but unfair to those afflicted. However, it is the burden we, CF people, will bear and each in our own way, will beat down. If you are physically able to persevere after each thorn stick, and if you are strong enough in mind and body to climb the stem, the flower, like life, is worth the effort.

Obviously, I can't remember the physical trials I went through those first two years of my life. Aside from those early CF-related complications at birth and those first two or three years, I didn't have too many complications as a young boy. Therefore, I will pick up my *climb* and fight from my teenage years.

I was told as a young boy I had cystic fibrosis but really didn't know the impact it would have on me until my first hospitalization for pneumonia as a young teen. *In home* nursing and self-medicating didn't exist at the time, so hospital stays of two weeks or longer were not uncommon.

These hospital "stays" consisted of early morning therapies, IV meds, and blood draws followed by mid-afternoon therapies, IV meds, and blood draws. Guess what the night's itinerary was. Numerous other tests done day and night were thrown in just to break up the monotony. I have literally had hundreds of X-rays and do not understand why I don't glow in the dark.

As a patient admitted for a serious regimen of IV therapy to combat lung infection, I would somehow still find time to stroll up and down the hospital halls. With IV pole in tow, I would visit my fellow patients as soon as I felt well enough to. My hyperactivity had mellowed a little (or at least that's how I remember it), but I was probably still going like the Energizer Bunny.

At that time, in the late sixties and early seventies, hospitals still allowed CF patients with active infections to room together and mingle with each other on a daily basis. As a matter of fact, they actually had a *day room* where they encouraged the kids to gather and play games together. Back in the late sixties and early seventies, there was still little known about our lovely disease. For instance, how easily transferred bacteria and viruses can be via physical contact and through the air. After all, families with more than one child with CF have no choice but to expose the children to each other. Since the percentage of children born with CF to a couple both carrying the recessive gene is 25 percent, it was fairly common for families with multiple children to have one or more with CF.

After making it through the first few days in the hospital with high fever and acute congestion, I would make the most out of each stay in Long Island Jewish Medical Center. I remember Dr. Gorvoy telling me how pleased he was and how important it was for me to be as energetic as I was. I don't seem to remember the nurses being quite so happy about it. Having my doctor tell me that being active was a good thing, resonated with me and still does to this day. Aside from my coughing fits, occasional hospitalizations, and shortness of breath with activity, I was basically like any other adolescent my age. I had hobbies, loved sports, and had raging hormones.

Lisa's Room

Lisa's room was three doors down from mine on the fourth floor in LIJ. The fourth floor, in the main hospital was where Dr. Gorvoy kept all his CF patients—pediatric and teens. There really weren't many patients with CF over twenty at the time, so it was basically children and young teens on that ward.

Lisa was about fifteen, one or two years older than I, and very cute. She was not a shy fifteen-year-old by any means, and perhaps, she was even more forward because her mother was a high level employee at the hospital. She had a surgical procedure done on her leg a few days before I was admitted and was to be bedridden with a cast for a week or so.

As I was making my rounds as four north's personal entertainer one afternoon, Lisa and I began to talk. At some point in the conversation, she mentioned that I was cute. Now, I was already aware of that, but hearing it from this adorable blonde confirmed the high opinion I'd already had of myself. Have I mentioned yet that I was vain as a young man? With that, she told me to come back to her room at one o'clock in the morning to *visit*.

Now, patients are encouraged to mingle and meet in the day room, but to my surprise, not to sleep together. So when the *graveyard shift* nurse, Bertha, entered the room at about three in the morning, finding me lying next to Lisa, I was pretty sure CF wasn't going to be the cause of my demise. Bertha was a very large woman, and when she explained how inappropriate this was, I decided to agree with her. While I was afraid Dr. Gorvoy would get wind of this, along with being very embarrassed, Lisa got a good laugh out of it all. Little more than a kiss was transacted, but I'm fairly sure that when I told my friends the story, there were some embellishments involved.

Looking back on that night, Lisa not only made me feel special, but also contributed in keeping my spirits *up*. What she probably didn't know is that in her own way, she helped me in wanting to meet more girls just like her...oh yeah and to keep fighting.

Trying in Vein

LIJ is a teaching hospital with colleges and universities from all over the world sending their students for medical training. As a patient, quite often you will see medical students either participating in or observing the initiating and administering of intravenous medications and numerous other procedures. Keeping in mind for most of these future doctors, nurses, and technicians, this is their first experience working with real patients, and as one of those patients, a high-level of tolerance is required on your part. Due to the multitude of hospitalizations I have had and the respect I have always had for doctors and nurses alike, when it comes to patience and tolerance, I have developed a high threshold.

This threshold was tested during one hospital stay in 1971 when I was introduced to a young group of trainees from Texas. The seven students along with the head technician gathered at the foot of my bed. My permission was asked for and given for one or two students to try and start up an IV line, which was requested by Dr. Gorvoy.

Unlike today's IV syringes, these needles were only about an inch long and made of nonflexible relatively thick gauge steel. That is to say, a stick from one of these was the equivalent of a painful bee sting or worse. For those of you who were unfortunate enough to have this done to you back then, you get my meaning, and you have my sympathy.

The first two or three rookie technicians were done trying, unsuccessfully of course. Pain and anger is starting to set in early in this episode as I am very congested at the time and running a fever. I am still composed though when the technician asks me and then pleads with me to allow another student to give it a try, then another, and still another. After the seventh stick results in one more gouge of my muscle and failure to access the vein, *eureka*, my threshold peak had been reached. I recall almost involuntarily grabbing the heavy IV pole with full bags of antibiotics contributing to the weight, picking it up, and almost throwing all of it out the fourth floor window. How and why I didn't, I still don't know.

After the trainees disappeared quickly from the room and a few minutes passed, the head technician put ice on both of my now, swollen arms, and waited. An hour later, my IV was inserted by the technician in about ten seconds. The CF amusement park is full of fun rides.

Outside Looking In

As a teen, nothing was about to stop me from enjoying my life, least of all cystic fibrosis. Despite the delightful experience with the young guns from Texas throughout my life, I often volunteered to participate in various trials and studies pertaining to CF. Like most teens and young men in their twenties, I felt I was indestructible. Though the severity and increase in my lung infections persisted, I never really felt my life was in jeopardy. Little did I know at the time, it was.

When my sister Valerie passed away, a very harsh reality was staring me in the face. Oddly enough and perhaps due to the faith I had in my own strength, this reality never really shook me. I felt then and continue to feel as if I am on the outside looking in at someone else's life unfold. I may not be able to give a definitive reason why this is, but I'm sure feeling this way has had a huge role in my survival. It's almost as if my psychological makeup won't allow me the thought of possibly dying from this damnable disease. This feeling is not something I try to or even can control. It saves me from having to work at staying positive in the face of all the sickness I've endured.

This sense of indestructibility I seem to feel, for better or worse, is something I wish I could share with all those terminally ill. I am not naive in thinking that all those with terminal illness will live longer than their fate will allow if they share in my feelings regarding death. I believe it has more to do with my fear of not being here to enjoy life, and it's my defense mechanism against dying. Perhaps the rebellious feelings and anger I have toward CF has fueled my motivation to continue fighting and not allow it to beat me.

A Variety of Laughter

Through junior and senior high school when I wasn't battling pneumonia, clearing my lungs out in the nearest bathroom, or sitting in the classroom, I would play as many sports as I possibly could. My grades were decent in school, but I was always more interested in physical activities and entertaining.

I loved my high school years and never wanted to miss a day for fear of missing something exciting or funny. So much so, I would often go to school with fevers and nasty infections just to be there. As a junior and senior in high school, some of my teachers would let me do a bit of *standup* comedy if the lesson was completed and time allowed. First, you should know that I am perhaps the worst joke teller in the world. I am one of those people that get about one sentence away from the punch line and starts cracking up. So I will tell you why, in spite of this, I am certain I missed my calling as a standup comedian. I don't make this claim with arrogance; I make this claim with confidence.

I am in awe of comics with quick wit. Don Rickles (if you are on the younger side of life, you probably haven't heard of him) was and still is one of the funniest and quick-witted comics to ever live. Robin Williams is also one of the best improvisational comedians there has ever been. I am fairly sure neither of them has ever told an actual joke from beginning to end.

As a result of this outstanding talent, as I boasted earlier, I was voted wittiest in my graduating class of 750 students. I'm sure Mom would have been slightly more impressed if I had been Valedictorian *and* wittiest of my class, but there you are. I just love to make people laugh, and I could and would go off about anything.

My biggest regret in life is not using my quick wit to pursue comedy as a career. I can't even say not returning to college after having to leave due to illness, and working instead, was as big a regret as not going after my dream. If I could do it over, I would make that dream come true.

This brings to mind a particular dream I had one night while sleeping in Harrah's Casino in Las Vegas years ago. The running joke with my family and friends is about how *lucky* I have been regarding just about everything in my life. Sarcasm, my friends, can be an effective comedic release for me, but you've probably realized that already. At breakfast the following morning after this dream, I felt the need to let my sisters and mother know what goes on in my mind behind closed doors and under the covers. So this is how luck, and the mind of Richie Keane works:

I find myself now on an airliner, cruising at about 33,000 feet when the captain announces there are serious problems with the engines and the situation is grave. As all on board begin to get nervous and are approaching panic mode, I stand up tall and demand everyone's attention. I am very loud and their undivided attention is achieved. In a much calmer voice, I make the suggestion that instead of all out confusion and screams of terror, we might consider a different approach in handling this situation.

Since we won't experience any pain or broken bones after the inevitable crash, why not use the thirty seconds or so we have left and treat our last moments as if we are on a giant roller coaster. Everyone put their hands way up in the air and yell, "Weee!" This will be so much fun, won't it? My fellow passengers do so.

This is how the reporter on the scene described it: "Tragic crash as an airliner goes down over the desert. We have a report now, that all on board have mercifully perished instantly…no…wait…I'm now getting a report there is a lone survivor. Yes, we are told that despite having broken every bone in his body, Richard Keane, as he has been identified, unfortunately never lost consciousness. However, when our reporter asked for an interview, she was told by the doctors that this wasn't possible. Mr. Keane seems to be in a strange sort of shock. With both arms broken, he just sits on the hospital bed, raises his arms straight over his head and yells, "Weee, weee," over and over." Oh, what a lucky man, he was. Welcome to my world, and mind, readers.

One of my favorite memories as a senior in Baldwin High School was our class variety show. This was a comedy show basically, where skits were put on for the parents, teachers, and students of Baldwin High School. I was fortunate to be part of a pretty closely knit senior class. I don't remember much trouble at all within the class as far as fights or bullying went, which is pretty impressive for a class as large as ours in 1974. We were more concerned with making the most of high school, academically, athletically, and spiritually. Some of us—ahem—leaned more toward the spiritual aspect of it. We all decided to put on the best variety show Baldwin had ever seen. Of course, we all think we succeeded.

So the variety show was my time to shine, and I wasn't going to waste my opportunity to make a few hundred people laugh. I loved being in front of an audience and found it a very comfortable place to be. I realized at a young age that I can actually entertain and make people laugh for a while, and this was very fulfilling for me. That's what I was meant to do and unfortunately lacked the foresight and direction to perhaps achieve success at that profession. Regrets, I have a few.

Motion Emotion

While in high school, I played football until I was a senior, had my own intramural basketball team, and played baseball until I was a sophomore. I was always the lightest guy on the team in football, but I played running back and defensive back for six years during my youth. Football was always and still remains my favorite sport to play and watch. I've been a bowler since I was a child and when I was in my twenties and thirties, I participated in numerous tournaments while carrying a 190 bowling average. I'm a decent golfer, play a little tennis, and until I turned 40, played twenty five years of softball as an above average pitcher. That's right, above average, now that's vanity.

A skier since age seven, I am envious as I watch all these kids snowboarding now and wish it was around when I was young. It looks like a blast, and I know I would have loved it. I am not boasting here, but instead, conveying how proud and fortunate I am to have been able to play this many sports in my lifetime. Especially because I know the odds were stacked heavily against me from the get go. As I mentioned earlier, I knew the more active I stayed, the longer I was going to be here. And by the way, I lied, I was boasting a little bit.

Those of you reading this who are my CF brothers and sisters, I will now give you the best advice I can possibly give you regarding our disease—stay as physically active as you possibly can. I'm sure this has been repeated to you many times over by your doctors and parents. I don't care. At the risk of being even more repetitive, stay in motion. Whether walking, running, or just doing some light sit-ups while watching TV, make it a point to get some exercise a few times a day. When you're not feeling well, I get it, it's not easy to stay active. This is why, when you are feeling about as healthy as you can, exercise your body. This will not only keep your lungs stronger, along with whatever muscle groups you're using at the time, but also will help loosen the mucus in your lungs. The other important advice I will give you all concerns that junk in your lungs, get it out and I don't care what it takes. I understand it's a difficult thing to do, especially in public. Too bad, bring tissues. I am convinced this is the main reason I am still on this planet.

Keep moving, you will feel better emotionally and live longer by staying in motion!

Group Cystic Fibrosis

Along with the increase of lung infections I incurred, during my mid to late teens, came the inevitable increase of medical bills for my parents. At sixteen, I began the process of applying for Medicare and Medicaid. For those of you that have been through this process, especially back in the seventies, again, I sympathize. This was not an easy or uncomplicated process by any means. From start to finish, about two years passed before all the criteria were met, and I was accepted for approval by the Medicare programs. Since the majority of doctors in the US didn't know about or hadn't really heard about Cystic Fibrosis in 1972, it stood to reason the government-run programs hadn't either.

Numerous letters from my doctors, mostly from Dr. Gorvoy, and a tremendous amount of help from my Social worker, Fran Belluck were required to complete this process successfully. Fran Belluck guided me through the channels and was truly a godsend in regards to this whole ordeal. An appearance before a county judge with tape recordings from my doctor explaining the disease of cystic fibrosis was mandated before they would approve assistance. When the smoke cleared, I was indeed eligible for Medicaid, and a small amount of supplemental security to help pay the bills. So as you can imagine, those two years were not the most enjoyable I had experienced and a bit harrowing and frustrating. I've spoken with some of the younger people with CF and they have told me the process of applying for government assistance programs is now a more expedient process.

It still drives me crazy, that even with insurance, the vast array of medicines, tests, and doctor visits I am relegated to, it continues to cost me thousands a year. I didn't request this disease, yet I must pay for the privilege of trying to endure it. Sensing anger, are we?

Fran Belluck always had a special place in her heart for Dr. Gorvoy's Cystic Fibrosis patients. The social worker in charge of all social services in LIJ for many years, until her retirement in the late nineties, Fran left a legacy of love and caring that I am confident is unparalleled in any other hospital system. Many programs still in place today were started by this special woman.

One of the programs Fran initiated was the teen CF group. This group was formed to give these young patients a forum to express themselves in any way they'd like, be it complaining about their illness, therapy procedures or anything else on their minds. As that group became a success with a relatively high patient turnout, the adult CF group was then formed. I participated in the teen group for a short while, but got more involved with the group as an adult.

As a result of years of research, the reality regarding how airborne germs and bacteria can be transferred from patient to patient, these groups could no longer be conducted. CF patients are so susceptible to lung infections, the frequent coughing taking place in these meetings proved detrimental to their well being. While these meetings were held, though, it was a bit comforting to know others were sharing some of the same issues you were dealing with. The internet is now loaded with CF chat rooms, and I have to believe trailblazers like Fran Belluck had a big hand in starting such forums.

John's Legionnaires

I met John while in my late twenties at one of the adult CF meetings. He was probably about thirty five years old at the time. John was very tall and thin but seemed to be in pretty stable condition for an older CF patient. This was very encouraging to me to see a man or woman for that matter with CF in their thirties as there weren't many that reached that age.

Statistics have shown that males with CF have a slightly longer life expectancy than females with the disease. I am not exactly sure why this is, but my guess would be that, overall, males are more apt to work out and often will continue to play sports into their twenties and thirties. Generally, this will make them somewhat physically stronger than females and perhaps that extra strength allows them to fight a little longer.

John was a twin who had lost his brother to CF a few years before we met. He was a very intelligent man with a degree in computer science. John and his wife had just recently adopted two little Korean sisters. He was doing his best to live a good, meaningful life while, like myself, battling a difficult strain of our shared disease. Many hospitalizations were necessary over the course of his life, mostly for pneumonia, but some also for pancreatitis. We were able to discuss and compare notes on both of these problems, which proved to be therapeutic for both of us.

John and his wife would join me in attending the CF groups' annual picnic at Eisenhower Park in East Meadow on Long Island. Fran Belluck, of course, would organize various social functions for the group every year. Each year, it seemed we would lose one or two of the group to CF. It was a little strange and scary for me, when it came to befriending fellow CF patients, knowing that it was sometimes obvious I wasn't going to see some of them the following year. John was unable to play in any of the games with his legs and body so frail, but we managed to have a good time nonetheless.

I arrived at an adult meeting one night and was told by Fran that John was hospitalized recently with legionnaire's disease. He had been down to Atlantic City speaking at a seminar in one of the hotels and caught the disease through the ventilation system. I visited John one night soon after at LIJ Medical Center when I was given the okay to do so by Dr. Gorvoy. John's wife was with him when I arrived. I was shocked to see how thin he really was as he laid on his side in the fetal position with a pillow pushed between his bony knees.

We talked for only a little while, and although I was wearing a surgical mask, my visit had to be cut short due to the risk John posed to me. After the usual patronizing words one might say to a gravely ill friend, John spoke to me.

John spoke angry words then, and it stopped me in my tracks. This quiet gentleman was furious that after fighting cystic fibrosis all his life and trying to lead a productive life, legionnaire's disease will take him from his family. I had no response to that except to say MaryAnne and I loved him and were very sorry. What do you say to someone who knows they're going to die?

I thought of Valerie as I left the room. John died a few days after my visit. I used some of the anger John had displayed at his incredibly unlucky circumstances, as my own, to battle this disease. I have to thank Fran Belluck and John for helping through yet another round of my own fight with CF.

My Pancreas and I

I came home from college at age eighteen after one year of school, due to my initial attacks of pancreatitis. My pancreas was already diseased because of CF, and if it wasn't damaged enough, I completed the job while I was away at school. I want to make clear that I always went to classes while I was there and left with no grade less than a B+ for the year. That being said, I could possibly have gotten by with a few less beers, etc. The "etc." is added because after all, it was the seventies. I've always felt kind of lucky to have been a teenager during the decade of the seventies. The music was awesome, especially if you liked to dance and it seemed as if for those ten years a perpetual party was taking place. Enough said.

For those out there who have had the pleasure of suffering acute pancreatitis, my sincerest thoughts are with you. Pancreatitis is an inflammation of the pancreas that affects some, but not all, CF patients. Thick mucus in the pancreas blocks the pancreatic ducts and disrupts the flow of pancreatic enzymes. This blockage of the pancreatic ducts creates two very basic but very large problems.

Without sufficient amounts of pancreatic enzymes, normal digestion of food is impaired and therefore, physical growth in general is interrupted. Supplemental enzymes in the form of capsules called Creon are taken with food to assist in the digestion process. The second problem is, with the ducts blocked and not allowing a normal flow of enzymes, pancreatic atrophy can occur. This is the main reason for the acute pain I suffered with pancreatitis.

With any amount of food taken into the stomach while the pancreas is inflamed, an attack of pain ensues. Enzymes begin to work on digesting the food, and this activity alone disturbs the pancreas. As is the case with many diseases, pancreatitis does not affect all patients with the same degree of severity.

I was diagnosed with acute pancreatitis and was hospitalized immediately after returning home from college. I dealt with the intermittent pain, severe more often than not, over the next twelve years.

To describe this pain is to ask you to imagine being doubled over or in a curled up position as someone pushes a rock the size of a softball into the middle of your abdomen just below the ribs, as if they were trying to push it out the other side. This results in a pulsating pain, which for me, was often excrutiating. When one is in the middle of one of these bouts of pain, everything must come to a halt and your focus can be only on the pain. The times when the pancreatitis attacks became unmanageable at home, I would be admitted through the emergency room at LIJ.

When I first experienced these attacks, the pain could be controlled relatively well with some extra strength Tylenol and a warm compress laid on my abdomen. Eventually, the throbbing pain became so severe that the pain killer Demerol had to be used.

As is true with any narcotic, the more one is given the drug, the more dependent the body becomes on it for relief of pain. Doses have to be increased over time as the body builds this resistance to the drug. When I was first given Demerol in my late teens, I thought it was the best thing since Led Zeppelin's "Stairway to Heaven." Fellow rock and roll lovers can appreciate the reference. I would go to the emergency room doubled over and in tears, and five minutes after the shot was given to me, I was on a stairway to heaven—no pain, only calm. Eventually, I came to despise Demerol as I would always associate the drug with pain and lingering nausea.

I recall one emergency hospitalization for pancreatitis when the ER doctors inserted a stomach tube down through my nose to pump out any bile or other fluids to see if this procedure would give me any relief. I expressed my concern as to what would happen when I cough up thick mucus and it becomes lodged between the tube and my throat. Wouldn't I choke?

Let's see if you can guess what happened about one an hour after the tube was inserted. As I was choking on the mucus and unable to call out for help, panic set in and I proceeded to tear the crazy glue like tape that was holding the tube to my face, off, and pulled out the entire tube through my nose. I still have dreams about that whole scene, and these dreams never end pleasantly.

As I approached thirty, these pancreatitis bouts occurred more often and became more difficult to bear. At one point, the gastroenterologists performed a procedure whereby they insert a stent to try and open up a relief port for anything that might be in the gall bladder or pancreas to pass through. Of course, my body rebelled against this stent. White blood cells attacked, infection ensued, and I then spiked a fever of 105. As delirious as I felt from this fever, I will never forget the agony of being laid on an ice bed for hours until the fever broke. That was not a good memory by any stretch of the imagination. The stent was then removed. Oh, well, *that* didn't work; next!

Soon after the failed stent, it was determined that a partial pancreatectomy was necessary to remove the atrophied section of the pancreas. When an ultrasound (sonogram) was performed on me as part of my pre-surgical procedures, the doctors spotted what appeared to be about six stones in the shriveled up, atrophied tail of the pancreas.

When the surgery was performed and the tail of the pancreas was excised, sixteen tiny stones were removed. Prior to the surgery, I overheard one young doctor outside my room saying he thought I was calling for pain medication to get high and not for the pain. After the removal of the many stones, this doctor came to see me and apologized for his comment. Everyone makes mistakes. The very next day, or so it seemed to me, the pain I had lived with for all those years was no more. Thank you to that surgical team for helping me to continue winning my bout.

Working the Stick

I began working at the Hewlett Inn, a bar my family owned, in 1973, the year before I went away to college. When I returned from school and recovered from my initial battle with my pancreas, I returned to work there full time. This decision to go back to bartending was a blessing and a curse. The main reason this move was a blessing for me was that a barroom can be a great venue for creating laughter and character, and laughter has always been something I've craved. The fact that I made very good money bartending didn't hurt either. The curse, well-being around all that smoke probably didn't help my lungs get any stronger, and being around all that booze, believe it or not, did not make my pancreas any healthier.

My father would call it, *working behind the stick*. The stick was another word for the mahogany bar I stood behind. I was a good listener, very personable, quick on my feet, and I could have given Tom Cruise a run for his money flipping glasses and bottles. Hope you all get the *Cocktail* reference. These shining qualities, along with being funny as hell, made me a successful bartender. The money I was earning at age nineteen allowed me to move out of my mother's house and support myself.

In this day and age, for any young adult to move out of their parent's home before age twenty-five seems to be rare.

With eight brothers and sisters, lack of privacy became an issue for me, so I made the move. I always got along with my siblings, so that was never a problem, and I actually loved being around all of them.

I never told my mother this, but years later, I felt somewhat guilty about not staying longer and giving her some money each month to help out. I know she would never have asked, but it is a small regret I live with. She could have used the money, and I certainly could have afforded it.

I received a phone call early one morning in 1984. It was my mother with the news that my father was killed in a car accident. I mention this now because it was at a time when I was considering some major changes in my life. The death of my father threw me for a loop and sidetracked me for a while. My father was only forty-nine years old and because my death before his was always assumed, it made me contemplate my own mortality. Obviously, my father didn't die of natural causes, but it still was kind of surreal for me. This particular scenario, him going before me, never entered my realm of thought.

I loved my father dearly, but unfortunately, had lost a tremendous amount of respect for him after finding out that in 1975 while I was away at school, he was having an affair. My older sister and I were very angry about this, and we both, in our own way, let him know this. My heart was broken over this. As a matter of fact, while making friends with other students at college, whenever "family" would come up in conversation, I would boast about how close my very large family was.

Mary Lou and I would both eventually be able to deal with the situation. My seven younger brothers and sisters would each, in their own way, have a more difficult time adjusting. My sister Valerie, at this juncture, was in a steady decline, health-wise, and my mother already had her hands full raising all of us for the most part, by herself. Mom would do the best she could, trying to explain to my younger siblings what was happening, but each of them were basically on their own trying to adjust to the situation.

My father was the type of man who was a great guy to be friends with. He was a handsome man and had a vibrant personality that people were drawn to. He was not, however, a good father when it came to taking part in raising his children.

When I was a young boy, I do remember some semblance of a *normal* family setting. Dad going to work, an occasional new car, beach days at Point Lookout and vacations once or twice a year up in the Catskill at the family's house. Unfortunately, as soon as he partnered with a friend in owning a Tavern a few towns away, that as they say, was that. Parenting was no longer a priority for Dad, and maybe it never was.

After a number of years passed, my mother, knowing of his affair, made him an offer he couldn't refuse, and he left. While she worked two jobs and barely made enough to pay the bills, he gave her very little money to help with the cost of living a large family will incur.

When I was a young boy, I used to believe the sun rose and set on my father, so you can imagine how saddened I was to find out he betrayed my mother and all of us.

I became very angry with Dad while Valerie was hospitalized during the last months of her life. He almost never visited either one of us during our hospital stays, and we for the most part, accepted this. We both knew he did not handle anyone's illness well. Some people don't; we both understood that.

During Val's last few months prior to her passing, my father had promised her one night he would come to visit. She had the nurse's aide, Pat Donnelly, bathe her, wash her hair, and make her as pretty as she could be. Pat was a blessing to have as an aide on four North at LIJ. She loved my sister and me and did everything possible to make Valerie's last two years as enjoyable and comfortable as she could. That night, my father never showed. My sister was very saddened by this, to say the least. I know my father loved her, but in my heart, I will always have trouble forgiving him for not seeing her that one last time before she died.

Years later, he finally tried to do the right thing by my mother, sending her some money now and again and taking out a small life insurance policy in her name. He also was taking classes and soon would be testing to become a court officer. He began making the effort of contacting his kids to try and have some sort of relationship with them. He also began to reduce his drinking to a minimum, which I personally was proud of, but maybe more amazed than anything that he had done so. Ironically, as he was in the midst of trying to straighten his life out, he was killed.

I don't think my father deserved to die because he neglected his wife and kids or for his poor choices in life, but sometimes, I think God said, "Sorry...too late."

This may seem ironic, but I need to thank my father now for the many life lessons I learned while bartending and for letting me exercise my wit while working *the stick*. I also think my brothers, sisters, and I learned from his mistakes and have made us all better, more caring people and where it applies, better parents. I sincerely believe he has helped us all along those lines.

You most likely did not set out to do that, Dad, but thanks. What's that they say...God works in mysterious ways?

Paying it Back

I happen to be a staunch believer in the old adage "What goes around comes around." As I wrote earlier, my father's death at the relatively young age of forty-nine seemed a bit harsh as a punishment for the selfish mistakes he made. The car accident that took his life, I believe, was a form of payback for the hardships he had put my mother through. There had to be a price to pay for not helping her out financially or otherwise during those rough years.

Payback really *can* be a bitch as they say. I have had a couple of things happen in my life that have strongly reinforced my belief in payback. Let me preface this by telling you there are some things I had done earlier in my own life that I'm not proud of as I believe most of us have. Someone else might look at the things I'm referring to and say they are not serious enough to put as much thought into and have as much regret about having done them as I do. I often think that some of the suffering I've gone through is payback for those poor decisions. I'm too old to change my attitude regarding the penance we each have to serve for negative decisions made during the course of our lives. So there you are.

Payback can also be *more* than a bitch for some people, especially for those who bully their way through life. There is now, and has been for a while, a positive movement in this country against bullying. The media's awareness and acknowledgement and the recent public recognition of this problem have been too long in coming. Classroom, workplace, and societal bullying need to be brought to the forefront and appropriately addressed and punished. As a young child, I was fortunate to have never been bullied. I hold real empathy for those children who were because to live in fear everyday whether on your street or in school is certainly a tragic existence. Emotional scars will almost always be left on a child that has been bullied.

While I was attending junior high school, there was a boy who, for whatever reason, was not fond of me. He wasn't one of the toughest kids in the school but was bigger than I (which was not saying much) and wasn't a friendly sort by any means. Let me make it clear that I was never touched by this kid, but the terror I felt for one whole year in seventh grade was real. He would threaten to kill me, beat me up, and whatever else he could come up with to frighten me. I had many friends and they all reassured me they wouldn't let him touch me but seeing and hearing this kid threaten me everyday kept my fear of him alive and well intact. Believe it or not, I survived seventh grade unscathed. Time passed and about six or seven years later, a friend of mine told me that this bully who ruined much of my first year of junior high school joined the merchant marines and drowned while scuba diving.

Seven years later, I was bartending in Peaches Pub—the local watering hole—when someone, probably a bit older and definitely a lot larger than I, followed me into the bathroom and began to harass me for no reason. While in there, one of my friends, one of my tougher friends, entered and suggested we finish the conversation outside. I convinced my friend to stay calm and not start anything, and he did, which in itself was a victory.

While we were outside, the situation was beginning to calm when the troublemaker's friends pulled up in their cars across the street. Upon seeing his buddies, his "whiskey" muscles swelled up again, and he resumed trying to instigate a fight with me. Before any fists were thrown, one of his friends called him over to the car. The road the man ran across to get to his friends was the town's main road, so you probably can guess what happened next.

This young man was only ten feet away from me when he was hit. The driver never stopped. I was the first one to get to him, and I screamed out to call an ambulance. An ambulance was not needed.

I am certainly not saying both of these instances of bullying toward me deserved a payback of death, but it does make me ponder. Perhaps, God thinks I have enough on my plate, and Richie Keane is not the person you want to harass or bully for no reason. Apparently, for some bullies, there will be a huge price to *payback*.

How About a Drink?

It wasn't until I was about twenty-six years old that I started to get a little tired of the fast life, which bartending was. I had seriously thought of going back to school to achieve a degree in physical therapy. Realizing I wouldn't be going anywhere in the near future, like heaven or hell and surprisingly, was probably going to reach my thirties, returning to school became a serious consideration. The aggressive deterioration of my pancreas was also an important factor in deciding to begin winding down my bartending days. However, I continued to work *the stick* for roughly three more years. Still have to pay the bills, you know.

Although the severity of my lung infections and pancreatitis attacks worsened from my late teens through my late twenties, I continued to stay very active. Between playing all the sports I loved and running my dogs, my physical activity never waned.

Unfortunately, also never waning during those early years was my alcohol consumption. Two factors contributed to this problem. The first is fairly obvious. I worked in a bar, a place where alcohol was easily accessible. The second is that alcoholism and addiction is in my DNA as it is an inherited disease in my family.

My father, grandfather, and some other relatives in my genetic line were alcoholics, and I had my own issues to deal with along those lines.

It is fair to say that between the ages of seventeen to twenty-nine, I pretty much beat the hell out of my body with alcohol and everything that goes along with growing up in the seventies and early eighties. I rarely drank before 7:00 p.m. On my work nights, though, it wasn't long after seven that I'd have my first one. For a person predisposed to alcoholism, it was difficult for me to be disciplined enough not to indulge. I make no excuses, I always made the conscious choice to drink, predisposed to alcoholism or not.

I do, though, have many great memories of those years. Ski trips, softball tournaments, and dart matches, all sponsored by the different drinking establishments and restaurants I worked in, were a tremendous lot of fun. Those twelve years were a big part of my life, and many of the experiences I had during those years contributed in molding me into the person I am now. I can certainly admit I should have had better control over the amount of drinking I did, but I like the person I have become, so I don't regret the years I worked behind the *stick*. Life really is too short to live on other people's expectations. We can do anything we want provided that we will be responsible for the consequences, and most importantly, we won't regret anything.

There were other factors contributing to the lifestyle I led and enjoyed until I reached thirty. I was blessed to have had good and caring friends over the course of my life. All of my friends have always been understanding and supportive of me. They were all aware of and observed me deal with my health issues daily, always offering any help they could. My close circle of friends from high school all did pretty well academically, and today, thankfully, all of us have good jobs or careers.

The problem was just about everything we did as a group back in high school and then in our twenties revolved around alcohol. I am not complaining, mind you, just stating a fact. This involvement with alcohol didn't seem unusual to us as all but two of my five or six closest friend had at least one parent who was an alcoholic. Drinking or *partying* was the norm in our families and was near impossible to get away from at the time.

When we get together now as men approaching our sixties, we laugh at how we were totally aware of the fact that we were alcoholics at that time but just accepted it. We actually would call each other up and say, "Hey, you wanna go drinking?" Of course, this only implied one thing, and it wasn't about having one or two cocktails while we socialized and talked politics. We were a happy group of guys that only wanted to have a good time. We never caused trouble, so what was there to get away from?

The alcoholism in each of our families combined with growing up in the decade of the seventies was a volatile combination. As for myself being of Irish decent, having an alcoholic father who owned a bar, well, you complete the thought. By the way, only one or two of my close friends drink at all these days, and the couple that do never overdo it. I am very proud of my friends for fighting through the difficult disease of alcoholism within their families and coming out the other side stronger, healthier, and better people for it.

I think that speaks volumes about learning from your parent's flaws and not emulating them but instead, making a change to better, and in my case, perhaps extend your life. My friends—they know who they are—because of their love, strength, and sincerity, are directly responsible for helping me get through my own bout with drinking.

Alcohol is also known to partially or fully nullify the effect of some oral antibiotics. For the most part, whenever I knew I was going to have a drink, I made it a point to take my pills hours before then. Of course, there were times when it was unavoidable, and I would have alcohol in my system along with the antibiotic. It is due to *those* times that I sometimes wonder how I made it out of my twenties alive at all. Sometimes, we are *all* too human and will use poor judgment resulting in poor choices. I have been fortunate to have lived long enough to learn from the consequences of my choices.

During one of my hospital stays for a pancreatitis attack, Dr. Gorvoy walked into my room and made it very clear he was not at all content with the way I was conducting myself concerning my alcohol intake. This was the first and only time I ever saw him express anger toward anyone, and unfortunately, it had to be me.

I was about twenty-seven years old at the time of this little meeting we had in my hospital room, and I will never forget it. He very firmly explained to me that if I kept abusing my pancreas the way I had been, it would be too diseased to function at all. Therefore, I wouldn't be able to digest, and I would die. I did cut back quite a lot but didn't stop completely until a couple of years later. Thick as a brick sometimes, I am.

Outside of a couple of drinks, I allowed myself to celebrate New Year's Eve, 1999, and an occasional sip of a champagne toast at some weddings; I don't drink at all. I tell people if they ask why I don't have a drink with them that I drank enough in my twenties and took an advance on alcohol for the next fifty years.

Prednisone and Pulmozyme

In the 1960s and '70s, aside from oral and intravenous antibiotics, aerosolized medications were introduced as a new form of treating serious lung infections. Back then, a plastic tent was set up over the patient's bed and the medicated mist would be pumped by a compressor into the tent and breathed in by the patient. This mist helped to break up the mucus in the lungs, so when physical therapy or postural drainage was performed, coughing up this mucus became easier. Most of the time now, instead of the tent, a mask or plastic mouthpiece is used so that the antibiotics and other solutions are inhaled directly into the lungs with only a small amount of mist or medication escaping.

In my lifetime, numerous advancements have been made in the therapies and medications used to treat CF. One of the more successful medications in aerosol form used to help clear the lungs is Dornase alpha or Pulmozyme. Again, unlike those born with healthy lungs, cystic fibrosis patients are missing an enzyme that helps to thin the mucus lining the lungs. Pulmozyme is an enzyme supplement that is in liquid form and is inhaled twice a day with a nebulizer. A nebulizer is basically a small air pump or compressor to which tubing is connected, leading from the pump to the mask or plastic mouthpiece to be used by the patient.

This inhalation is followed by intense postural drainage. This drainage therapy involves someone cupping their hands and with an alternating cadence, pounding on different areas of the upper body of the patient. There are now vibrating vests patients wear to achieve the same result. The inhaled meds and the drainage are an effective way of causing the patient to cough, loosen, and rid themselves of the mucus. The more mucus one can get rid of, the better chance one has of not allowing infection to get a foothold. Inhaling antibiotics is not quite as effective as having it flow directly into the vein via IV but generally more effective than taking the meds orally. Unfortunately, not all antibiotics come in aerosol form.

Prednisone, a corticosteroid, is an anti-inflammatory and immunosuppressant medication introduced around the mid-1950s. Most people reading this have probably heard of prednisone or know someone personally who is using the drug. It is given to people suffering a number of different ailments. For CF patients, it is an effective way of helping to reduce inflammation and open up the bronchial tubes and airways.

I remember the first time Dr. Gorvoy prescribed prednisone for me. He was very optimistic this drug was going to help me and all his patients breathe much easier. Prescribing the proper dosage for each individual patient was still, for the most part, a trial and error process. Looking back, I was given what would now be considered a fairly high dose, for my size and weight.

The steroid worked well on me and served the purpose for which it was intended.

The side effects of prednisone as with other steroids are many and when taken for long periods of time can be life-threatening. This steroid not only breaks down muscle mass and bone, but profuse sweating, steroid-induced diabetes, bloating, weight gain, and hemoptysis (coughing up blood) are not uncommon side effects. Steroid-induced depression can also occur. I had the good fortune to experience all of these. Please excuse my sarcasm. In this particular instance, I am using sarcasm in lieu of frustration and anger.

For cystic fibrosis patients, prednisone, with all of its side effects, is still the most effective way of inducing less strenuous breathing by reducing inflammation and opening up those airways. Fortunately, for most people taking prednisone, there is a point reached where they can either discontinue taking the drug, or be prescribed minimal amounts. Unfortunately, for us CF people, periodic use of prednisone can be effective for a time, but eventually, as the disease progresses, continuous use of the steroid is required. As end stage cystic fibrosis approaches and one is then fortunate enough to have had their lungs transplanted, small doses of prednisone will be taken continuously post surgery for life as an immunosuppressant.

MaryAnne

I met MaryAnne Anzano while we were juniors at Baldwin High School in 1973. Our respective circle of friends, though coming from different junior high schools, had much in common and quickly merged into one very large circle of friends. After my first conversation with MaryAnne, I knew she was a sweet, kind, and compared to me, an extremely quiet girl. We soon became good friends and would talk together about everything. It wasn't long at all before I realized she understood more about my health situation than most.

To this day, I really don't know why after just having met MaryAnne, it was so easy to tell her about all my problems, health, and otherwise. She was a calming influence on me at the time, I guess. I respected that as I was not easily calmed. Little did she know she would be listening to and participating in any and all of my many problems for many years to come. She would have to wait about thirteen years, though, from our first meeting to hop aboard the *joy ride* called Richie Keane.

Soon after I introduced MaryAnne to my mother, it occurred to me they have some personality traits in common. Both are conservative, bright, and unlike my father and I, do not like to draw undo attention to themselves.

MaryAnne and I were still just good friends at the time, but while I was dating other girls, my mother would ask me from time to time why I wasn't dating MaryAnne. If I remember correctly, I responded by saying something to the effect of, "Why would I subject this sweet girl to the likes of me?" We remained very good friends throughout high school.

MaryAnne went to Hartford University in Connecticut and earned her Masters Degree in Special Education at Adelphi University in New York. Just to stress once again the kind of person she is, MaryAnne has been teaching children with learning disabilities now for thirty-four years. The patience required for teaching at any level, let alone children with special learning needs, is patience that I cannot fathom. This, to me, speaks volumes about the content of her character. While at the University of Hartford, MaryAnne organized and took part in various charity functions benefitting cystic fibrosis.

While we were away at school, MaryAnne and I, along with some other friends, would occasionally visit each other at our respective campuses. The year, I was away at Sullivan County Community College in upstate New York, MaryAnne and a couple of my good friends from Brockport and Oneonta Universities came to visit and celebrate my big eighteenth birthday.

This was a big one for me for a couple of reasons. One, because of what my friends had heard about CF, they weren't sure I was going to make it to eighteen, and two, back then, eighteen was the age one could legally have a drink. Turns out, I had been practicing for my eighteenth for about a year or so prior.

It was early in that first year away at school that my pancreatitis reared its ugly head. My birthday is November 2, so I hadn't been at school long before the pain began. With my friends going out of their way to come celebrate with me, I figured I'd have a drink or two just to ease the belly pain I was having. That's my story, and I'm sticking to it.

Close to the end of the school year, I returned home to be admitted to LIJ Hospital with pancreatitis. I had completed all my courses at school and had only to take my finals when I left. The dean of students made a nice gesture when he told me I could take all the finals at a later date due to my circumstances.

As time passed and years went by, MaryAnne and I kept in touch only periodically. She graduated Hartford and remained in Connecticut to teach for the next seven years. For myself, I made some good choices and some bad choices over those same seven years. MaryAnne would later tell me I was *sewing my wild oats* as they say, and I guess she was waiting for the thread to run out. Maybe she knew me better than I knew myself.

I was working at our town's premiere watering hole, Peaches Pub, one night in 1985 when in walks my friend MaryAnne. We hadn't seen each other for a good six years, but we talked and laughed as if we had been out together the night before.

It was a little awkward for me to do this, having been good friends all those years back, but I asked MaryAnne out to dinner for our first official date. The fact that she was driving the coolest car on the road at the time, a 1984 Mazda RX7, and was sporting a beautiful new nose job, didn't hurt. Please know I am kidding. Personally, large noses never bothered me. As a matter of fact, Barbara Streisand and Cher, in my opinion, were two of the sexiest looking women to me, in their prime, of course. My wife should have stuck with the "original," but she's happy, and therefore, I am.

Get me to the Church

I've joked with family and friends all of my adult life about just how unlucky I am regarding my health, gambling, and just about everything else. Of course, I make light of what I've been through and continue to go through to get a smile or a laugh out of them. It does make me a little crazy sometimes that the health problems don't seem to, and apparently will, never end. However, if I'm going to complain about not having things go my way, when things do go my way, I must acknowledge that also. So, I will tell you, the night that MaryAnne walked into the pub to see me for the first time those years ago, was not only the luckiest night of my life but the night my life was changed forever.

By the time I turned twenty-eight, I had gotten out of the pub scene and was working as a bartender in a very popular restaurant a few towns away. I knew it was time to wind down the bartending scene and calm my lifestyle down. MaryAnne was not thrilled I was still working late into the night at McClusky's Steak House, and she made it her job to let me know this once or twice an hour. In 1986, MaryAnne's older brother asked me to come work for him in his photo lab. Working on a computer half the day and making job deliveries the other half was a nice change for me after twelve years of what sometimes seemed like a perpetual happy hour.

In February of 1988, I was once again admitted to LIJ for acute pancreatitis. My pancreas was so diseased and inflamed by this point that any food or liquid, bland or otherwise, would trigger an attack. After going through the usual process of fasting for a day or two, my pancreas would calm down, and the pain would subside enough for me to be released. After this particular hospitalization though, I wouldn't be going straight home.

After this discharge from LIJ, I would be driving straight from the hospital to the church MaryAnne and I would be married in. I have always been a very punctual person and would not be late to the altar. Though I was still a bit weak and pale, the wedding ceremony and the reception went on as planned and were amazing. Coming straight from the hospital to the church on our wedding day was just a sample of what the adventure of being married to me would entail for MaryAnne.

It was just one month after our wedding when I had the surgery to remove the atrophied tail of my pancreas. Thank God that thirteen-year-old pancreas ordeal had finally come to an end. On February 6, 2013, MaryAnne and I celebrated our twenty-fifth wedding anniversary. Because of the love, patience, and care she has always shown me from the day we met, I was here, alive and kicking for it.

Alana and Lara

At seventeen, I was tested at LIJ to see if I could one day be able to father children of my own. I guess it would be more appropriately put to say I *tested* myself. I had been practicing this grueling test for a number of years prior, so I passed with flying colors.

The complications caused by CF to the reproductive system combined with the vast amount of certain antibiotics given me since birth rendered me impotent, or so it was thought at the time. I was told there was only a one percent chance of me causing a pregnancy. So I was *shooting blanks* and would never father my own child. For me, as a young man, the fact that I couldn't cause a pregnancy was the only, and I mean the only positive thing to come out of having CF. Indeed, I was promiscuous as a young man and the result of that sterility test suited me just fine.

Within the past twenty years, medical procedures have been introduced whereby the man's semen can be extracted and by using the in vitro method and impregnate a woman. This was an important breakthrough for young men with CF wanting to start a family with their own DNA. For many years, this wasn't the case.

Shortly after MaryAnne and I were married, we discussed the possibility of having a child by way of adoption. We eventually decided against it for two reasons. First, the reality was that we didn't know what the near future, let alone the distant future held for me regarding my health. Obviously, I didn't want MaryAnne to have to raise a child alone should I become irreversibly ill. Secondly, MaryAnne had just moved down from Connecticut to start teaching in New York and needed to get established in a new school district and continue her career. Having a child at that juncture of her life wouldn't have been prudent.

One year prior to MaryAnne's relocation to New York, her younger sister, Toni Lee, gave birth to a baby girl, Alana. MaryAnne and I were spending a great amount of time with Alana during her visits down from Connecticut. Her sister had just opened up a restaurant with her husband and found it difficult to spend much time with Alana.

We both love kids, so MaryAnne and I took Alana just about every weekend and often on weeknights to *hang out* with us. Three years later, Alana's sister, Lara was born. I will tell you that the relationship I have today with Alana, twenty-nine and Lara, twenty-five is as close as any parent can have with their own children. I never will have my own children, and I feel extremely blessed to not be unfulfilled in this area. I cherish them both. They are incredibly beautiful young women inside and out.

The times we spent together on vacations, driving around, looking at Christmas lights, or just sitting on the floor talking are times I will cherish much more than they will ever know. Hopefully, they will read their uncle's book and realize that as much effort as I put in to help mold them into who they are—amazing young women, they helped me much more than that in becoming a better man.

Spending as much time as MaryAnne and I did with the girls certainly wasn't in our plans as we started our lives together, but being such an important part of these girls' lives has had a big role in my continued drive to live and fight this disease. My fear of not being able to watch these girls grow up because of CF was real but unsubstantiated, thank God. Thank you, Alana. Thank you, Lara. I will love you both forever for giving me even more reasons to fight for my life.

Tyler's Choice

Schneider Children's Hospital, part of Long Island Jewish Medical Center, was built in the mid-sixties. The cystic fibrosis clinic, pediatric oncology, and the neonatal units were all relocated from the main building of LIJ and housed in Schneider's soon after construction was complete.

Dr. Gorvoy had all of his patients, young and old, requiring hospitalizations, admitted to the third floor of the new hospital. As I was approaching twenty years of age, my first few admissions were a little weird, sharing a floor with children much younger than I. This bothered me a little, but not too much. Some other older patients were not as comfortable with the arrangement and requested rooms in the main hospital. Fortunately, or I should say unfortunately, there were almost always one or two CF patients around my age on the floor during each of my admissions. This made it a little more comfortable for me while on the unit. The nurses were all trained specifically to know how to treat and deal with CF patients' needs, and most were extremely thoughtful and personable.

Often, I would see the same patients admitted during my frequent hospitalizations. You must remember, back in the late sixties and early seventies, there were not nearly the number of CF patients there are now. This, of course, is disappointing news.

I first met Tyler while we were hospitalized together on four North in the *old* hospital at LIJ. I'd say we were both about ten years old at that time. We got along well and hung out in the day room together whenever we were able to. He was not nearly as thin as I and looked to be in very good shape. He was also a little better looking than me and that I did *not* like. Excuse me, but I'm the center of attention here on four north, or didn't you know that?

After that one hospital stay with Tyler, about ten years would pass before I would see him again. Perhaps, he was able to keep his lungs in good condition or was just a little luckier than I. Whatever the case, we always seemed to miss each other during our CF clinic visits and respective admissions.

Together again years later in Schneider's Children's Hospital, Tyler looked even healthier and more handsome at twenty-one years of age. A Harley Davison guy who loved riding his motorcycle, Tyler sported a Fu Manchu mustache, looked much older than I, and if I didn't know him, I would have thought he was the model used for the infamous Marlboro man. All of my life, until about ten years ago, I always looked a bit younger than my actual age, so I wasn't too upset that he looked like a full grown man, and I could have passed for his son...almost.

Tyler seemed to me, a quiet sort who kept mostly to himself while in the hospital. Of course, I would have none of that, and when we both started to respond to the meds given us and felt a little better, I would engage him in conversation. I've loved motorcycles ever since I was a kid and loved listening to Tyler talk about his riding excursions and the various bikes he owned. Personally, I never owned one, and in hindsight, it was probably better that I didn't, but I did always have the desire to have one.

Tyler did not look like most CF people. Most CF patients I knew had a distinctive look to them. I do not mean this in a demeaning or mocking way, just making an observation. For those experiencing difficulty with the disease, having a somewhat hunched back, clubbed fingertips, and thin frame are basically common physical characteristics of the CF person.

The hunched back look and clubbed fingertips are a result of that person struggling to get oxygen into the lungs. One's back may become hunched due to the continuous physical action of expanding the lungs and chest to the max so that the individual can inhale and take in as much oxygen as possible while he or she is struggling to breathe. After time, this constant struggle to breathe will leave the person's chest cavity at full expansion at all times, hence, the hunch in posture. Expansion of the chest and lungs for maximum oxygen intake is why you will see marathon runners, athletes, and just about anyone out of breath—bend over to breathe. The action of just bending over expands the chest and lungs, and one is able to breathe easier.

When a person is having difficulty breathing or even gasping for breath, the heart works overtime to send oxygenated blood to the lungs and body. For the CF person, this constant, strong flow of blood pushes out toward the body's extremities (fingertips and toes) and over time will cause those extremities to have a bulbus look to them. Although my back is slightly hunched from my own struggles with breathing, I have never really displayed a very pronounced CF *look*.

Tyler had none of these traits and looked amazingly healthy to me. Looks, as we all know, can be deceiving. Tyler was admitted to the hospital this particular time for a pneumonia infection and hemoptysis. Hemoptysis is a condition where bleeding occurs in the lungs due to infection, or the rupturing of blood vessels due to intense coughing.

Tyler, to my amazement, was also a cigarette smoker. This amazed me because early in my teens, I tried to inhale smoke from a cigarette once. If I remember correctly, it was actually a law back then that when you turn sixteen you must, to be labeled *cool*, try smoking. The smoke I inhaled made it half way down my throat before I coughed it out. I can remember thinking, *How could anyone inhale this thick smoke, let alone someone with a lung disease?*

I've personally experienced mild episodes of hemoptysis over the course of my life, but thankfully, these episodes never became too severe. My sister Jenny has had some more difficult issues than I with bleeding in her lungs. Thankfully, her numerous bouts with hemoptysis have been controlled and stopped fairly quickly.

Tyler had a serious, ongoing battle with his hemoptysis. It doesn't take a genius to figure that smoking didn't help his cause, but as you read further, you will see Tyler was pretty set in his ways. Years passed and it had been quite a while since I had last seen Tyler. Another attack of pancreatitis brought me into Schneider's once again.

After two or three days of being bedridden with pain, I was finally relaxed enough to take some walks up and down the hall. There Tyler stood, much thinner than I had last seen him and hooked up to a portable oxygen tank. His skin was ashen, and he wasn't looking well at all. We talked for a few minutes only as standing and talking was enough to exhaust him and leave him gasping for breath.

Dr. Gorvoy came to see me early the next morning as he always did on his rounds. I never made it a habit to ask about other patient's situations and problems, but I told him I was shocked to see Tyler in that condition. Since my sister's death, Dr. Gorvoy, at my insistence, was always brutally honest with me about everything to do with my disease. He explained to me that the more severe cases of hemoptysis are very difficult to get a handle on. Constant pneumonia infections complicate the situation and make it almost impossible to control.

No real successful trials or methods of treatment for this severe a case of hemoptysis had been successful around the time of Tyler's case. Boston Children's Hospital had come up with a method of controlling the bleeding that was showing some bit of promise. Tyler was transferred to Boston and experienced slight improvement. He wasn't coughing up near the amount of blood and with the addition of strong doses of vitamin K, which helps the blood to clot, included in his regimen of medications, the bleeding could be stopped temporarily. Tyler's numerous and increasingly severe lung infections were another issue entirely.

His lung capacity was deteriorating rapidly at this point in his life. Transplants, though not nearly as advanced as they are today, were being performed at a couple of hospitals on the east coast by this time. Dr. Gorvoy told me in our discussion concerning Tyler that he was definitely a good candidate for bilateral lung transplantation. However, like all transplant candidates, he must go through an extensive battery of tests before he can be declared eligible. This is time consuming and can be exhausting.

About a month or so had passed before I was back for a routine checkup with Dr. Gorvoy. I asked how Tyler was and if he had gone through the transplant surgery yet. He told me Tyler decided not to have a transplant and wanted to let nature take its course. I wasn't capable at the time of getting my head around that decision.

How could he not want to fight and give himself as much time as possible? I then asked my doctor how Tyler was doing regarding the hemoptysis. Dr. Gorvoy then told me Tyler passed away two weeks after I had seen him last in the hospital.

I'm older and somewhat wiser now, and I understand we all have to make our own difficult decisions in our lives, even when the decision you make affects your own mortality. Rest in peace, Tyler.

Ribs, Anyone?

My body has remained strong enough to endure much in my fifty-six years, and I am grateful for that strength beyond words. Not only was I blessed with the physical ability to stay active, I was able to play some fairly strenuous sports up until two years before my transplant. I actually was still bowling and bowled a 660 series (you bowlers know that's a great series) with the oxygen tank close by until just a few months prior to the surgery. Thank God I rolled a lot of strikes because throwing two balls in a row was a bitch.

After making a full recovery from my pancreas surgery in 1986, I was able to return to all of my sports leagues. I even set a personal record for myself one day in 1989. Playing eighteen holes of golf in the morning, pitching both games of a double header in softball that afternoon, and bowling three games that Sunday evening is something I am very proud of. That will never happen again and that's okay. The fact that I was able to accomplish that at thirty-three impressed and maybe even surprised Dr. Gorvoy.

My new lungs are stronger, thankfully, than my lungs were then, but now, I'm a bit tired after playing one full round of golf. After all, I am a fifty-six-year-old man trapped in an eighty-six-year-old body, or at least I feel that way occasionally. I still bowl, but softball has been over for me for a number of years due to the brittle bones with which I am now blessed.

My disease resume increased by one in my early thirties when steroid-induced osteoporosis made its first appearance. The first rib fracture I suffered occurred while I was playing softball. I went into a shoulder roll or somersault after catching a fly ball and felt a pop in my chest. I knew right away, without ever having had one, that it was a broken rib. I've broken other bones, as most of us have, but to those of you who have had ribs broken, I think you'll agree, it's a whole different animal.

The pain involved with this type of injury is magnified with each breath you take. I would have to get used to that pain in a big hurry. Since that first cracked rib, I have endured at least thirty more either cracked or broken ribs. Some of the cracked ribs were what are called linear fractures, meaning a split along the length of the rib. Most have occurred while having intense coughing fits. Some multiple fractures have occurred occasionally during a single fit. On other occasions, just a hard, single cough would do the job. Still, other ribs have broken with light to medium pressure put on my chest or back.

Just for fun, here are a couple of examples of how brittle prednisone has made my bones. While at work one day, my back felt a little tight, so I asked one of my waitresses to gently crack my back. This girl couldn't have weighed more than 115 pounds. She wrapped her arms around me from behind as one does to crack a back and started to apply pressure...*pop*.

As I was riding in a golf cart one day out on the course, I spotted a baseball cap the group in front of us had apparently dropped. Being the thoughtful person I am, I pulled up to the hat, leaned over the side of the cart to pick it up, my chest pressed slightly against the armrest...*pop*. One more and I think my point will have been made.

One night while lying in bed, the TV remote fell on the floor as will happen from time to time. While remaining in the horizontal position, I leaned over the side of the bed to retrieve it. Just a little pressure put on the ribs...*pop*. Oh, come on now, really?

Two factors contribute to the difficulty those with cystic fibrosis who acquire osteoporosis have to deal with. First off, the pain from a cracked or broken rib can be intense for anyone. When harsh coughing fits are added to the equation, you can multiply that pain times ten at least. While I am in the midst of one of these coughing attacks, I would have to get into what I describe as contortionist positions to do my best to alleviate the pain. Depending on where the crack or break was located, determined what position I would try to achieve. On most occasions, I would have time to prepare for the coughs and attempt to achieve these positions as I could feel the congestion rumbling in my chest. Other times without warning, I would suddenly, involuntarily cough hard. I won't even describe *that* pleasant feeling to you or it will start to sound like I'm feeling sorry for myself, and I probably am.

The second and more dangerous problem the CF person with osteoporosis and broken ribs has to deal with is infection. The intense pain caused by rib cracks and breakages inhibits one from taking strong, deep breaths. Because it is so painful to take an actual deep, lung filling breath, coughing and clearing the thick mucus out of the lungs becomes extremely difficult if not impossible. Consequently, the mucus remains and festers in the lungs and airways. This can and most times will eventually cause infection. With all of my rib injuries, this particular scenario was all too common for me. Prednisone and its wonderful side effects, what are you going to do? As they say, some things you can't live with and you can't live without.

Port to Port

Sometimes, we have to be grateful for the small things that make our lives a little easier. If I had a dime for every time an IV line was started on me, well, you know the rest. In the early nineties, the many lung infections I had endured up to that point in my life began to take their toll on my veins. The vast amount of IV lines and various other needles used for injection and blood draws left my veins hard and rubbery. This hardening of the veins made it very difficult for the doctors and technicians to access them for IV needle insertion. Finally, Dr. Gorvoy had the team surgically insert a port in the upper right side of my chest.

This quarter sized, half inch thick aluminum sphere sat just under the skin and was connected to a ten-inch micro tube running through one of my veins. This small advancement in medical science was one thing in my life I was extremely grateful for.

The port has a small rubber center into which the needle that delivers the antibiotic would be inserted. Ports will last in your chest about five to six years before they have to be removed, primarily due to infection at the site. My first port lasted in my chest for six years. The less a port is accessed, the longer life it will have for the patient. For normal blood work, the arms and hands must still be used to get an accurate reading of the blood samples. The needle used for the port is a much smaller gauge needle than those used for IV, PICC, and Midlines.

These port needles are so fine, when they pierce the skin, usually only a small pinch is felt. Peripherally Inserted Central Catheter (PICC) lines are temporary IVs also surgically inserted in the arm and threaded directly into the right atrium of the heart. These are generally used when the patient is expected to be on IV meds for at least a month.

Midlines are thick gauge needles with six to seven inches micro tubing that are inserted peripherally, threaded into the vein, and can be painful to have put in if the area around the "site" is not numbed sufficiently. These IV lines can generally last up to one month.

Having one of these midlines put in was the only time in my life I ever came close to fainting from the pain of a needle. Two nurses and a technician came to my home one afternoon to start up one of these midlines. I learned that memorable afternoon, the techs are only allowed three tries at accessing a vein for midline insertion per each patient.

The first two tries obviously didn't succeed or I wouldn't be telling this *painful* story. As they entered my skin for the third try, I was praying silently, as I am pretty confident they also were, for a successful conclusion.

The pain from all the digging around they did finally got to me and, without any alcohol at all, I felt a little drunk and lightheaded. I didn't quite pass out, but the techs, after the third failing try, had to call it a day.

Off to the hospital I went for surgical insertion of the line with local anesthesia. I believe I insisted on the anesthesia at that point. When one is prescribed IV medication for long durations, or periodically for the rest of their life, the port is obviously the preferred choice. My second port was put in the same day my first, which had gotten infected and was taken out. This second port, inserted in my upper left chest lasted a number of years and was removed during my transplant. Again, sometimes we all have to be grateful for the small things in life.

Sugar, Sugar

Slightly amazed myself that I was still here at forty, I didn't have to wait long to realize my fight with cystic fibrosis wasn't near over. Just prior to my pancreatectomy at thirty, I was informed that due to the condition of my pancreas, I would become diabetic at around forty. The damaged and diseased pancreas, combined with the heavy doses of steroids I had been given during my late thirties sealed the deal.

Eureka, I turned forty, and approximately, fifteen minutes after midnight of that November second, I was diagnosed with type 2 diabetes. My response to the doctors ten years earlier when first told the good news about my diabetic future was something along the lines of "whatever, how bad can it be…it can't possibly be as bad as CF." Good call, Richie.

Living with diabetes is not easy and has its own set of troublesome issues. Again, diagnosed a type 2 diabetic, I have been insulin dependent from its onset. No pills for me, thank you, let's go straight to the needles.

Testing blood sugar levels on a regular basis is one of the annoying routines the diabetic has to deal with. To be honest, I am not near as disciplined with the maintenance of diabetes as I have always been with CF. This is not something I'm proud of, just stating a fact. I've been diabetic for sixteen years now and basically know if my blood sugar is high or low by how I feel. I don't recommend other diabetics gauge their sugar levels by how they feel, but I haven't yet had any major malfunctions because of diabetes. I'm fairly sure I will now, though, after *that* statement.

Of course, I jinxed myself with the "major malfunction" comment in the above paragraph. I am writing this particular paragraph approximately six months after that statement, and I now *have* had a major malfunction. This particular incident was a direct result of me taking this disease called diabetes too lightly.

I am an extremely punctual person in every aspect of my life, something which my loving wife is not, and it drives me crazy, but I digress. My routine during the work week is almost down to the minute. Take oral meds, shower, inject insulin, walk the dog, and drive to work has been my morning schedule for twenty-three years. Immediately after arriving at work each day, I eat breakfast. Granted, eating breakfast at 10:30 is not "doctor recommended," but there you are. This itinerary has worked for many years because no matter what schedule you choose as long as you are consistent, your body will adjust and you should be fine. What the diabetic should do every morning, which up until now I rarely did, is monitor his or her blood sugar. One particular morning, not checking mine, cost me dearly.

As I was in the middle of the fourth step of my routine, walking the dog, my blood sugar dropped radically in a short period of time. I was about a quarter of a mile away from home at the time and without candy or any type of food for that matter. This is not a good combination, and this is the reason why diabetics are always supposed to carry glucose tablets, candy, or orange juice on them at all times. I don't remember fully the last one hundred yards or so before I reached my house, but I do vaguely remember putting Abby in the basement, or so I thought. As I reached the landing at the top of the stairs, I reached for my cell phone to call 911, but it was too late.

I went down on one knee, and what followed was not only the most bizarre event in my eventful life but also the most dangerous. I fell face down and began to have violent seizures. These seizures, from start to finish, lasted anywhere from five to ten minutes. The frightening part of the whole episode was that for most of the time, I knew what was happening but was powerless to stop it. I had never "seized" before, so I didn't know if they would eventually stop, or this was how I was going to make my exit from this world. I seriously had those thoughts as I was periodically banging my face against the tile with the waves of convulsions that came and went. With all that I have had happen to me, before the incident, I never thought I was going to die as a result of what I was going through at that time.

I was frozen in the same position—right side of my head laying against the tile, both elbows tucked in at my sides, left knee bent up to my side—for the full duration of the event. With each wave of seizures, these parts of my body hit the tile floor with a force so strong, it was like I was trying to break through to the basement. Finally, the waves began to come further and further apart. Still unable to move from that position, I began to moan from the pain in my eye socket and knee cap as they had been playing the bongos on the floor for what seemed like an hour. I wanted to cry at this point but was unable to even do that. With no one there to help me, I was genuinely frightened of not being able to survive this. How much more tile pounding banging could my head take, and how was I not knocked out by now?

Another wave came, I moaned again and prayed, but my body remained rigid. I waited for the next wave, but it never came. Finally, my body went limp. I rolled over on my back and wiped the sweat off my face. I was aware that I still had to get sugar into my system right away. I got up off the floor, realized my right eye was closed and walked drunkenly to the phone and then made my way to some Hershey's Kisses.

My brother-in-law, Marcello, picked me up quickly and drove me to the nearest emergency room. I don't remember most of the ten minutes it took to get to the hospital, probably because Marcello told me I had a seizure in his car, and he was slapping me to try and snap me out of it. I remember looking at the ER sign as we arrived at the hospital but then proceeded to have my final seizure right there on the ground outside the ER.

I was told by the ER doctor that most people whose blood sugar drops below thirty-five will either fall into coma or have violent seizures and then fall into coma.

Now, this whole ordeal was obviously my own fault, not having glucose tablets or candy on me to raise my sugar level. However, once again I felt as if I was on the outside looking in at my body, paying the price of not being diligent in checking my blood sugar levels that morning. And once again, I would not allow any thoughts of not surviving this episode of my life. *I* will decide when my time is up.

When I was finally stabilized intravenously with D50, a dextrose solution, I was visited by my wife, Marcello, and our friend Colleen. What happened next was a perfect sign of the times we live in.

Before they made it over to my bedside to hold my hand, give me a kiss, and console me, all three took out their phones and began to take photos (they knew by then I was okay). When I finally was shown by Marcello what I looked like, I understood the paparazzi like action all three of my loved ones took. I looked as if a purple baseball was surgically attached to where an eye once was. Let's leave it at that. Two things I will always do from here on out—take a reading of my blood sugar every morning...and always have glucose tablets or candy on me.

The CF person with diabetes does have other important reasons to keep his or her blood sugar levels under control. Lung infection or any infection for that matter will take longer to heal with unstable blood sugar levels. Broken bones will also take longer to mend with erratic sugar levels. When I was first told this little fact, I did start to be more vigilant with my sugar and carbohydrate intake. I visit my endocrinologist four to five times a year and my long-term blood tests (readings for the three months prior) have, for the most part, been stable. I'm sure the fact that I am on my feet and active for a good part of each day helps to keep my blood sugar in check.

I see my kidney doctor once or twice a year as I have come to find out that kidney damage is a common occurrence among diabetics. As a matter of fact, not until shortly after my transplant did I find out that lung transplant recipients often will require kidney transplants down the road. The combination of diabetes and certain medications taken by transplant recipients, because they are passed through the kidneys can, over time, cause serious damage to those kidneys. Of course, the better control one has of his or her diabetes, the less probability of kidney damage occurring.

Uncontrolled diabetes can also be responsible for serious heart problems and disease. Aside from having high blood pressure and hypertension, all of my heart-related tests have had passing grades so far. The only difficult issues I am dealing with as a result of having been diabetic for this many years is neuropathy and diminishing eyesight.

Diabetic neuropathy is most common among people who have had diabetes for ten or more years, patients that don't have good control of their blood sugar, and older diabetics. Neuropathy is nerve damage in the feet and or hands. I developed diabetic neuropathy in my feet about two years ago in 2010. It can be quite painful at times as it feels like electric shocks occurring in different parts of your feet with each step you take. At rest, for me anyway, the pain is minimal to nonexistent.

While I am at the gym, the shocks I get in my feet while on the treadmill can get severe enough to stop me in my tracks. Diabetics do have to maintain some discipline in foot care if they are to minimize these related problems. With advanced neuropathy and poor circulation, it can eventually become extremely painful to walk at all. With poor care of the feet and blood sugar neglect, serious infection, such as gangrene can set in. If not taken care of and treated properly, amputation may become necessary. I don't want to sound too morose here, but I do want to explain to readers who may be at risk for this disease, that diabetes is not something to be taken lightly. With the neuropathy I now have, I have learned this the hard way.

Over time, diminishing vision is always a concern and eventual inevitability for anyone with diabetes. For me, trouble with my eyesight while reading did become an issue for me about seven years after I was diagnosed. Since then, every two years or so, I've had to switch to stronger lenses to read comfortably. My vision, as far as distance is concerned, is only now, after fifteen years with diabetes, becoming an issue.

A diabetic's ongoing loss of vision, as with all the consequences associated with the disease, is slowed by diligent control of one's blood sugar. Although my long-term tests on average show more than adequate control, these many years with diabetes are definitely taking their toll on my sight.

Any time a new problem with my health has arisen, I've fought that problem with defiance, anger, and without fear. However, I will admit this, and I have to this day never mentioned it to my wife, the thought of going blind scares the hell out of me.

A Session of Depression

Depression, thankfully, has never been in my repertoire of diseases or disorders. There have been though, many times it would seem the problems I had were piling up and non-ending, and my sullen mood would reflect that. I was fortunate to never fall so deep that I couldn't climb out.

I do know people, some very close to me, who have some mild depression issues and also some who have to deal with the more serious, manic and clinical depression. Panic attacks, which can go hand in hand with certain types of depressions, are frighteningly real for those experiencing and struggling to live through them.

Up until Christmas morning in 1998 when I awoke to a frightening new world and for the five weeks that followed, I could never, as all those who have not experienced clinical depression, really understand what this disease entail.

Something wasn't quite right when I awoke that morning. I hadn't been sleeping well for weeks prior and was given Ambien to remedy the problem. To some extent, this medication had a reverse effect on me. On more than one occasion, I was totally unable to sleep while under the influence of Ambien. I was also feeling very weak; as for many weeks prior, heavy doses of prednisone were taking their toll and weakening my muscles. This *cocktail* of medications combined with the lethargic mood I had already been mired in was not a good combination. My lungs were free of infection at the time, so it was concerning to me as to why I was so weak and lethargic.

Let us discuss the wonder drug, Prednisone, once again. Most people, I would imagine, have heard about mood swings associated with people taking steroids. Perhaps, *roid rage* is a term you may be familiar with. Basically, whether one is injecting steroids to increase muscle mass or taking steroids orally, a dangerous chemical imbalance within the brain can occur. Prednisone had already been part of my medication regimen well before 1998.

Corticosteroids, like prednisone, help reduce inflammation of bronchial tubes in the lungs and again are crucially important drug treatments for those with lung and breathing problems. Unfortunately, with prolonged use of high doses of prednisone, neurotransmitters in your brain are adversely affected. These neurotransmitters are blocked and unable to send the proper signals to other parts of the brain. The chemical in your brain that controls emotional balance, serotonin, can be lowered to dangerous levels. This drop in serotonin levels can bring on mild depression in some people and in others, plunge them into major clinical depression. Can you guess, once again, which category I fell into?

Anxiety and panic attacks, crying uncontrollably for no reason, thoughts of suicide, and the fear of losing one's mind are just a few of the symptoms clinical depression can bring on. It would be weeks from that Christmas morning before I could leave my house without fear. Panic attacks and intense fear ensued whenever I was left alone for any period of time.

The description I give those who ask about how this episode of this depression affected me goes something like this: I would rather suffer through five double lung transplants and a year of nonstop acute pancreatitis than to repeat what I went through for that period fourteen years ago. If you happen to be a person who has had a lung transplant and pancreatitis, but *not* depression, you may think I am crazy for feeling this way. I will now do my best to explain what happened to me. I am not trying to frighten anyone here, but if you find yourself in a similar situation, perhaps this will help you better deal with the scene than I did

For the first couple of weeks, with holiday vacation time off from school, MaryAnne was home most of the time, thank God. When she did have to leave to go to work, I would watch the clock, cry, and basically freak out with paranoia until she returned home. I still wonder what my dog, Sheena, thought of the spectacle she witnessed everyday after Mommy left.

This panic got so bad that a couple of times, my mother and sisters would be called to come *babysit* their forty-two-year-old son and brother. I recall one afternoon being in such a depressed and panicked state that I lay, curled up in a ball, with my head resting on my sister Amy's lap. This lasted for hours while my mother and sister Mary Lou sat nearby, trying to keep me calm. Let me correct that, I should have said, trying to keep me sane.

I don't know exactly what time that morning I fell into the black hole of depression, but I fell hard, and it took awhile to climb out of this one. It truly seemed as if one minute I was reading the day's paper and the next I was a paranoid, frightened, uncontrollable crying mess. There really is no other way to describe the emotional state I was mired in.

I think about that particular day and others like it and wonder what my wife and family, who witnessed this firsthand, must have thought. This must have shaken them up as none of them had ever seen anything like it.

Perhaps the scariest part of the whole scene is that for every minute of that five-week episode, I was totally aware of what was going on. Why it was happening, and why I couldn't break out of it were questions I needed answers to ASAP.

Dr. Martin was the chief psychiatrist of LIJMC at the time of my session of depression. On a quick side note, the only *advantage* of being a lifelong CF patient at LIJ is that whenever any medical condition in need of attention arose, I was always seen by the chief of that department. I guess I've earned certain perks, being a lifelong member of the LIJ *club*. Two days after that morning from hell, Dr. Martin mercifully took me in as his patient. That was the good news.

The very bad news was that whatever antidepressant medication I was to be prescribed, was going to take approximately two to three weeks before results could hopefully be achieved. I've come to learn in my travels from doctor to doctor, and at present, I have thirteen, that in spite of all medical and scientific data gathered, many of the medicines prescribed for certain ailments, diseases, and disorders are still hit or miss, trial and error. This is in no way a knock on the excellent jobs my doctors have done throughout my life. I have been very fortunate in this regard. I am instead making the point that even with in-depth research and trials, certain medications will work better for some than for others.

After Dr. Martin explained what most likely caused my depression and anxiety, we discussed the various medications available to try and remedy the situation. Zoloft was the first antidepressant given me. To give the Zoloft an opportunity to work, a full two weeks was needed. All of these antidepressant drugs need time to try and raise the serotonin in the brain to normal levels.

Each day that had passed since the first day of my somewhat *out-of-body* experience was worse than the day before. I use the term out-of-body because in between the many episodes of panic, crying, and fear during each day, I felt almost as normal as I ever had.

I explained to Dr. Martin, while in these *calm* moments, I would tell myself, "Okay, everything's all right. No reason to be upset or afraid; let's just stay this way, and this can all be over right now." "Not quite yet, buddy," my mind would respond. I would then proceed to sit panicked, curled over in a ball or in the fetal position, and begin to cry. The fear and paranoia I felt at those moments, I cannot truly convey. This scene would repeat itself over and over for all of those five weeks with increased magnification during each episode. The doctor said that during these *states of mind* of clinical depression, my thoughts and actions were not uncommon.

I feel trying to describe what panic attacks and depression are to someone is analogous to attempting to describe what it's like standing on the ruins of Pompeii in Italy. I'm afraid you just have to "be" there to know. Zoloft, of course, failed to do the job after the allotted two weeks.

Near the end of the third week of my depression, hell, I began to entertain thoughts that I might actually be losing my mind. Looking back now, I think it was more like, "Oh my God, I'm losing my mind!"

I was desperate to stop what was happening to me and to stop the fear and sadness this was causing my wife. What could this episode of my life be doing to her?

As strong-minded and understanding as MaryAnne had always been with me regarding all of my health issues, my depression was pushing her to the edge. Her frustration and anger toward me and what I was going through was palpable and came to a head about three weeks into this insanity. I would be upset, crying, complaining, and with a facial expression of complete fear each time she came home from work. Going to school each day to teach her special education children must have truly seemed like a vacation for her during those five weeks.

Finally, I reached the end and had enough of it all. Against Dr. Gorvoy's and my wife's wishes, I insisted on going over to the psychiatric hospital, located next door to LIJ Hospital, for electroshock therapy. I was absolutely convinced at this point that I was going insane. We arrived at the hospital at 8:30 p.m., twenty minutes after they stopped accepting any more admissions.

I do not profess to be an overly religious person, although I do pray at night, but I feel God was looking over me that night, closing that hospital twenty minutes earlier. I had heard that some people are never quite the same after shock therapy. This isn't to say one can't live a normal and productive life post shock therapy, but I have heard stories of people that have had lasting emotional problems afterwards. Judging from the luck I'd had up until this point in my life, well, again, you finish the thought.

After the first two unsuccessful weeks of the Zoloft trial, Haldol, an antipsychotic medication, was introduced as the next course of action we would take to battle this depression. Haldol changes the actions of chemicals in the brain, trying once again to achieve normal levels of serotonin.

"Hopefully, two weeks after your first dose, you should have your life back," Dr. Martin said to me. Two weeks to the day later, I kid you not, I woke up and my nightmare was over, just like that. The relief and euphoria I experienced, I hope by now you can imagine.

To this day, I continue to take the antidepressant Wellbutrin, just as a precautionary measure. My doctor has weaned me down a bit on the dose and has told me I can stop taking it completely. I tell him and all my other doctors who ask me why I am still on Wellbutrin that I was so terrified by the experience I had, I feel a sense of security while on the medication. Whether this sense of security is false or not, and I know while taking Wellbutrin depression can still occur, as I will always be taking prednisone, is beside the point, it works for me.

Thank you, Dr. Martin, MaryAnne, and my family for getting me through those intense and frightening rounds of fighting. And thank you, CF, for continuing to keep my life anything but boring...I hate you.

ABCs of FEVs

My lung function started to decline fairly rapidly as I approached my early forties. It became apparent that I would have to face the reality of having to put an end to some of the sports I love to play. It had just become too stressful and exhausting to continue the pace I had been going at for so long. Not only were my lungs weakened by years of infections and the resulting scarring, the muscle mass in my legs and arms was deteriorating as a result of years of high doses of prednisone.

I realized even in my late thirties that my physical capabilities had already lessened significantly, but it still shocked me how quickly my lung capacity had begun to diminish. In the span of two years, when one goes from running at full speed around a baseball diamond, to not being able to walk at a good pace for twenty feet without gasping for breath, it can be a little shocking and depressing.

Dr. Gorvoy and I had spoken a number of times over those many years about the possibility that one day I would need lung transplantation. So it was that at age forty, when my Forced Expiratory Volume (FEV) 1 dropped down to about 35 percent, I was sent to New York Presbyterian Hospital (Columbia

University) to begin testing for eligibility of bilateral lung transplantation.

Basically, the FEV1 is the measurement of how much of your lungs are still able to take in oxygen, or to put even more simply, what percentage of your lungs are still working. The criteria required for transplant regarding lung capacity percentage has changed a bit over the years and for the most part, to be eligible for transplant, his or her FEV1 must drop below 30 percent.

The battery of tests I had to go through to prove eligibility was extensive, time-consuming, and sometimes exhausting but understandably necessary. After the few months needed for all departments of the hospital to gather and review their data, it was determined that I was indeed a good candidate for a double lung transplant.

I was not oxygen dependant at age forty when I was listed. Though the criteria for transplant regarding my FEV1 measurement was met, I was not in "desperate" shape, so I was listed but not activated. This was a bit confusing to me at first, but it simply meant my lungs were damaged and my breathing labored but apparently not labored enough to actually be eligible for new lungs.

If this sounds a little strange and confusing to you, you are not alone. As a matter of fact, this "activated" or "nonactivated" process of listing has since been done away with. Either you're eligible for transplant and will be called, hopefully at some point, or you're not. Shortly after I was initially listed at age forty, I was indeed activated for transplant.

One early morning in 1996, about 2:00 as I recall, New York Presbyterian Hospital called and told me to pack my bags; they had lungs for me if I wanted them. Originally, I was told that the waiting period for lung transplant could be months, or even years in some cases so I was caught totally off guard. I had only waited a couple of months when I got the call.

I immediately called Dr. Gorvoy and we discussed the situation....yes, at 2:00 that morning. I was only given fifteen minutes to respond to Columbia with my decision. After discussing the pros and cons of transplant at this juncture of my life, heeding Dr. Gorvoy's advice, I called Columbia and declined the lungs.

I could not sleep the rest of that night, mainly because I was kind of freaked out by the whole situation. I was also wondering, of course, if I had made the right decision. Let's face it, talking about receiving a new set of lungs and actually being called to the operating room for the surgery are two different things entirely.

As I look back the whole episode was a little overwhelming but exhilarating at the same time. Had it not been for Dr. Gorvoy's input and advice that morning, I fear I would not be here now to continue the process of annoying my wife.

To my surprise and delight, aside from the personal "depression era" I experienced at forty-two, for a couple of years during those early forties, my overall health, lung function, and even my FEV1 measurement stabilized somewhat. Congestion from CF was always present in my sinuses and lungs—that never changes, but pneumonia infections were occurring a bit less frequently for those few years.

I was able to work fairly steadily and even able to get in some golf, fishing, and other physical activities during that period of time. I pushed myself especially hard those years to stay in motion and took advantage of the times I felt I could exert myself. I would always take what I could get, physically, at that point in my life.

When it comes to lung transplant, the advancements made in the actual surgical procedure, post operation therapy, and anti-rejection medications can vastly improve in a ten year period. Life expectancy post transplant for the CF patient was significantly less in 1996, when I first got that life changing call, than it was then in 2007. So once again, my friend and doctor had been there for me at that morning in 1996, and once again he had given me more time. Thank you, Dr. Gorvoy, hardly seems enough!

A Goal of Life

Setting personal goals has always been an important driving force in my life and more importantly, my survival. This is not to say I've reached all my goals, by any means, but some of the more important goals I've set for myself have been achieved.

Reaching the ripe old age of thirty was a goal I had put out there for myself while in my mid-teens. At fifteen or so, having already surpassed, by a number of years, the life expectancy for a CF patient, shooting for thirty was pushing the envelope, and I knew it. Again though, my mind would not and still does not allow me the thought of dying before I feel my time here is done. After turning thirty years of age and having gotten through the whole pancreatitis ordeal, it was time for future goals to be set and pursued.

When I emerged from the pancreas surgery weighing in at about 115 lbs, my obsession (goal is too soft a word) became to gain as much weight as possible, as quickly as possible. I came to realize this is where having a good case of OCD can be your friend. I then proceeded to go after my goal weight of 150 lbs like there was no tomorrow...and I felt if I didn't put on some poundage soon; there might not be.

Complications with digestion and malnutrition are almost always an ongoing problem for a person with CF. It was for my sister Valerie as it is for me. We lack the enzymes needed to digest properly due to the mucus buildup in the pancreas as I explained earlier. To gain weight and to maintain that weight can be as frustrating as trying to lose or control your weight.

Protein and calorie loaded shakes are commonly prescribed methods to aid in weight gain. Advancements and improvements in the flavors and more importantly, the taste of these shakes have taken place over the years. When I first started drinking the various shakes the nutritionist recommended over twenty-five years ago, they were barely tolerable. They did slowly improve somewhat, and they were a big part of helping me reach that 150-lb goal, which, to be honest, I thought I would never reach.

It took a lot of shakes, pasta, pizza, and anything else I could get into my stomach to bring my weight up. Only two years had passed since I began my pursuit when my gluttony paid off, and for the first time in my life, I wasn't totally disgusted by how skinny I was. Reaching this goal was really an emotional moment for me as I had spent most of my life extremely self-conscious about my weight. I finally had what I considered (almost) to be a normal body to go along with my adorable face.

MaryAnne understood the importance of this moment and actually threw a surprise party for me with family, relatives, and friends. Seems a bit odd, celebrating the fact that someone stuffed his face for two years toward a "heavier" end. However, they all knew how frustrated I had been for years, and, they knew what a great guy I was, so we rejoiced together. (If you need to take a break now, I understand. I'm getting sick of me too).

I will always remember that celebration with fondness and the realization that MaryAnne was right. If I truly put my mind and body into any quest I pursue, I will succeed.

Like most people, I believe striving for the goals we set for ourselves, large and small, play an important role in our lives. I would guess there are probably only a handful of people in the world who have actually reached their full potential and realized all their goals in life. Most people will have failures and successes along the way, and I believe this to be healthy for the mind and soul. In my opinion, just the act of setting and striving to reach goals can be a positive driving force and motivation in some people's lives. It certainly has been and still is in mine.

For myself, recovering fully from that stomach surgery in 1988 was not just another goal set and reached. Considering the frail state my body was in at that time, to be able to recover and gain the weight I did and rebuild my body strength so quickly and significantly post surgery, was not only a goal, but a mammoth plateau reached in my life. In some ways, I felt more invincible than ever. If I was able to recover from that whole scene, nothing was going to take me down any time soon.

My confidence grew even stronger during my late thirties as I continued to defy cystic fibrosis. That confidence grew so that I now felt reaching forty years of age was not something to be "over" celebrated. Now I was beginning to get a little, shall we say, cocky, regarding how long I could survive this disease. Fifty sounded a lot more inviting to me at this point in my life than forty. Let's now make that our survival goal and shoot for that nice round number.

Through research and discussions with Dr. Gorvoy, I learned there had been some fairly significant improvements in bilateral lung transplants and more importantly, some progress with improving anti-rejection medications a few years before I was initially listed in 1996. It seemed every couple of years since the first CF lung transplant in 1988, new medications, therapy methods, and clinical trials were being introduced. There was growing optimism in the medical community about the future of lung transplants.

I also remember being told by the doctors during those earlier years, the longer I could live with my own lungs, the better off I would be when the time comes for transplant. So this became the most significant goal I would put out there for myself up until that point in my life….living to fifty years of age with my own lungs. Weakened and scarred as they were and having gone through all the other difficulties I had experienced, this would indeed be an amazing feat…if I do say so myself. I fought hard for that goal, and I made it so.

Now, six years out (lingo for how long post transplant patients have survived), I of course have set some new goals for myself. I'm not quite as cocky or confident as I once was about when my luck, or should I say, strength, will run out (I am also a realist *and* fifty-six years old). I won't get crazy and predict living until 2026, when I would be seventy, but I will tell you that I will still be on the internet, keeping in touch with old friends in 2016. We must have those goals to pursue! Thank you again to my wife, family, and friends for celebrating that much sought after goal of reaching the 150-lb mark with me. That achievement was huge, and may I never dip below that number again. Cystic fibrosis loses those rounds, big.

Three Little Ladies and a Man

I have been extremely lucky to have had three beautiful ladies other than my wife, help me to not only survive but enjoy and thrive during the last thirty-five years. Now, don't judge or think any less of me (if that's possible). These three ladies were born with four legs and fur. I had the good fortune and sheer pleasure to have risen from "puppyhood," Missy, Sheena, and now, Abby. Let me tell you a little about them.

Please don't ever underestimate the friendship, support, strength, and healing power having a loving pet and a pet to love can bring.

Missy was an adorable six-week-old German Shepherd mix that I fell in love with when I first eyed her at the rescue shelter. I was twenty when I got her, and we immediately began to train each other. She was an "apartment" dog, but we spent quite a lot of time outside. My days were free, as I was (living the dream) as a bartender in my twenties, so this proved to be convenient. No matter where I went or what time I came home, she would be waiting by the door with tail wagging.

I can personally attest to the fact that your pets can sense not only when you're angry or sad, but also when you're not feeling well. Whether I was in pain or feverish from infection, she would never bother me to go outside for her walk, as much as I know she had wanted to. When I returned home from my pancreas surgery, Missy was excited but careful not to bump me or get in my way as I walked gingerly around the house.

She saw me through many emotional and physical changes in the time we had together and although she probably didn't agree with all the decisions I made during those times, she never judged me. In retrospect, maybe I should thank God she couldn't speak. Missy lived thirteen and a half years and helped me through several big rounds in the "ring" vs. CF.

Sheena is the reason I should never have watched *Marley and Me*...I cried like an infant at the end of that flick. Labrador retrievers usually live to about ten to twelve years of age. I was fortunate enough to have Sheena for fourteen and a half years. Because of a lifestyle change, as far as working hours and personal behavior (ahem), I was able to have a much more structured relationship with Sheena than I did with Missy.

Sheena was a beautiful yellow Lab who, I swear, understood full sentences I spoke to her, not just one-word commands. This had been the case since when she was a puppy and then through adulthood. As a matter of fact, there are a number of people I have met, who would struggle to reach the same level of intelligent conversations as I had with this beautiful canine.

Yes, I am a dog person and I get that all of us "chosen" ones think we all have the smartest dog ever, so I will leave it at that.

Sheena was an incredibly athletic dog, as many Labs are, and this fact helped to keep me active and in shape. She, like Missy helped me get through some really difficult and harrowing times in my life. I always wanted a Labrador because I knew they were active, smart and, one might say, hyper dogs. I figured if we could combine our respective energies and as long as we didn't actually explode, we could help each other exceed our predicted life expectancies. This actually worked wonderfully for both of us!

Sheena was also astonishingly aware and sensitive to my emotional and physical demeanor. She was still a fairly active dog at ten years of age, but soon after we both started to show signs of slowing down. Our regular walks in the evening and our daily soccer games at the field were taking place less frequently. She knew I was beginning to show the effects of my illness and would lay by me during my nebulizer treatments and watch helplessly as the treatments would induce choking and coughing.

Sheena knew my limits and accepted them. Now, to be honest, had Sheena been two or three years old when my illness had progressed to where I was having more frequent pneumonias and nebulizer regiments, I am not sure she would have accepted my limits so readily. Had she been able to speak English, she probably would have said, "Stop shriveling up, and let's go the hell outside!"

To have Sheena with me by my side before and after my transplant was a blessing that I honestly can't describe to you. Aside from MaryAnne, she was truly the prime source of comfort for me during those life changing days. I have to thank my friend Sheena once again, as I did when I held her during her final minute of life, for helping me through my most difficult rounds in my life to date in my battle with CF.

MaryAnne and I discussed getting another dog after Sheena was gone, but we decided to wait a few years before doing so. However, only about one year passed when I started to get the itch for another four-legged friend. My significant other was not thrilled about it at the time and wanted to stick to the original plan.

I look back to one night about a little over a year after Sheena was put to sleep. Sitting on the couch next to MaryAnne, watching who knows what on TV, I told her she was my love, my friend, and my confidant...but I was lonely. I whined about being lonely just enough, or perhaps more than enough and my wonderful wife gave in. Now, after a few months of training this "energetic" puppy, I am very confident that either MaryAnne or Abby, and not CF, will be the cause of my demise.

Now Abby, *oh my God,* Abby. Some nights, if I listen real carefully, I can actually hear Missy and Sheena saying, "Good luck with that," while spinning in their graves. This beautiful, golden-eyed yellow Lab has come dangerously close; a number of times to having us legally change her name to Abby Bin-laden.

Abby is now a little over one year old and strikingly similar in looks and body type to Sheena. I experienced little to no problems training Missy and Sheena, and now I look back and consider myself very lucky in that regard. My first two dogs were quick studies as puppies. This dog Abby, makes "Marley" look like an angel. But, oh my God, do we love her. I'm pretty sure she is the most affectionate dog on planet Earth. Wish us luck…a lot of luck!

The reason I bring up and write about these "ladies" is very important for me to explain. It probably is already obvious to you that this goes well beyond being a dog lover. I am not just an animal lover but feel, as many others do, that some animals, especially dogs can be very therapeutic. Therapeutic, not only for those who are disabled physically, but also emotionally.

I was and remain still, extremely fortunate to have had loving animals by my side to support me through all my physical and emotional issues. Of course, people who love you and care for you can also be wonderful support systems, but when I am confronted with ignorant and insensitive people, as we all have been, the words I once read on a bumper sticker, "The more people I meet, the more I like my dog," rings true for me.

Because of the close relationships I had with my first two dogs, I often ask myself why I would subject myself again to the inevitable sadness and heartbreak I feel at the end of their lives. With Abby, if she lives to the average age for Labrador Retrievers, eleven years, I will be sixty-seven. I know that number is one that I will need all the optimism and strength I can call on, to reach. I *will* be there though, when it's her time, and

I will be sad...but I will also be very happy because I'll know she was taken into my home where she will have been loved and has had as active and as happy a life as did Missy and Sheena.

With Abby now, I sincerely and confidently feel I will live at least as long as she does, so I am looking forward to, regardless of what terror she puts me through these first couple of years, being here at least ten more years. Although my wife informs me that my continued existence on this planet is directly related to how long it takes me to fully train Abby Bin-Laden.

I love my four-legged lady friends and thank them from the bottom of my heart for their unconditional love and their important roles in keeping me alive.

Pleurisy

During the course of my life, when it came to dealing with the collateral, physical, and psychological issues and other problems associated with CF, I've always tried to be tolerant and brave. Bravery, fortunately or unfortunately, has never been a characteristic lacking in my personality. This is not a boast on my part, just fact. Perhaps, my bravery is a direct result of having dealt with much illness, many, many needles, and various other unpleasant medical procedures since I was very young.

In my mind, there isn't much that can happen to me in the "outside" world that can hurt me much more than what I've been through during my life. I haven't had much choice in the matter, so perhaps I've been kind of forced into being brave and tolerant. In any case, it is what it is.

The only medical procedure I have ever been frightened of is a blood gas. As far as my own personal array of illnesses go—CF, diabetes, osteoporosis, etc.— none of these scare me. They instead, anger me.

One's tolerance is tested continuously over the course of his or her life, we all know this. Once again, my own tolerance level was tested at age forty-five when another, shall we say spin-off disease of CF was added to my now, overflowing list.

Hot, steamy morning showers are one of the best therapies to help loosen the thick mucus, which is ever present, in the lungs of CF patients. It is especially important to do all you can to rid yourself of this crap in your lungs, especially every morning. This is because the accumulation of mucus is usually greatest after lying dormant for seven or eight hours. The pounding shower and steam, along with good hard coughing, is a great combination to rid one's self of this mucus.

One particular morning, after going through this routine in the shower and feeling for the most part, shall we say, phlegm free, there was still a rumbling and scratching feeling present in my lungs. I immediately assumed this was the start of an infection rubbing up against the ribs, which happens quite often with CF. With no fever present or an over excessive amount of mucus in my lungs, at least no more than usual, this feeling of scratching in my chest as I breathed soon became vexing to me. Basically, this annoying constant rubbing and scratching began to drive me crazy. After waiting a couple of days for it to subside, I began to get very angry when it didn't.

Something else to worry about, really? Are you kidding me? Off to the hospital I go to have my one thousandth X-ray taken of my chest. No confetti or balloons fell out of the ceiling though when I reached one thousand…very disappointing.

CF has now given me the gift of pleurisy. I'll certainly learn to deal with it as I really don't have a choice. I had heard of pleurisy but really didn't know what this condition of the lung was, what caused it, or what it entailed. I would soon learn.

A person's lungs are housed in their chest inside what's called a pleural cavity. This cavity is made up of two layers of membranes that separate the lungs from the chest wall. Normally, these membranes rub smoothly against each other as the lungs expand and contract with each inhale and exhale. When the surface of the lungs is inflamed, the swelling causes these membranes to now rub against each other resulting in the sensation of two pieces of sandpaper being rubbed together.

There are a number of reasons pleurisy can occur. In my case, rib fracture, followed by lung infection was the cause. At the sight of the rib fracture or infection, the resulting inflammation can be so acute that it pushes against the membrane lining and causes that friction. I was fortunate to experience only moderate pain associated with my bout of pleurisy. I've read about and heard stories of some patients that have experienced excruciating pain during these episodes. Looks like I got a bit of a break on this one

This went on for only a month or so, but that feeling of scratching and rumbling with every breath had succeeded in making me just a little more crazy than I already was. Thankfully, I've had to deal with this particular illness only once in my life, so far. That sound you here is me knocking on wood.

Tanking It

"You will *never* see me walking down the street, pulling an oxygen tank behind me!" This was the (long-winded) mantra I repeated for many years. I started chanting this mantra when I was about twenty years old. I had thought at the time that coughing and choking the way I did in public was embarrassing and disgusting enough. I certainly wasn't going to be one of those people walking around with an oxygen tank in tow and a tube sticking out of their nose. It's not that I lack sympathy for those in need of constant oxygen flow, although my sympathy lessens for those who smoked and are in need, but I personally find the sight of this oxygen tube disturbing and off-putting.

To say I was self-conscious about how I sounded while in the midst of a coughing fit is putting it more than mildly. Finding an alley, a bathroom, or some other secluded area became a priority for me when I felt a fit coming on. I often wish I wasn't the kind of person who let these personal, physical problems, none of which I can control, bother and embarrass me the way they do. For better or worse, these are some of my personality traits, and at this point in my life, those traits will never change, so it's out of my hands.

Perhaps now you can imagine how mortified I was, initially, when my lungs became so damaged and weakened, that I needed oxygen now and then just to get around. I got over being mortified about lugging the tank around pretty quickly, though. I realized unless I'm content sitting in one spot all day, I will need the constant aid of oxygen.

When I received my first delivery of oxygen tanks, it was a bit upsetting to me for a couple of reasons. First, the realization of the fact that my lungs were actually going to fail in the not too distant future, hit me hard, and second, I had not yet reached my goal of keeping these lungs until the age of fifty. I would have to keep these lousy lungs going for about one more year. You want a fight, CF? Try and keep me from my goal.

Although at this stage of my life I was dealing with serious breathing difficulties, some days were not quite as bad as others. Many people reaching end stage CF need oxygen around the clock. I must admit, I consider myself lucky in that respect. When I slept, I never needed that annoying oxygen tube wrapped around my ears. I was able to sleep surprisingly comfortably, right up until transplant time. I really was lucky in that respect. I slept well then, and I will never take sleeping without need of oxygen for granted.

However, when I did have to get up, whether for the bathroom or to clear my lungs out and cough, as soon as I began to move, oxygen was a necessity. Any mild activity, such as brushing my teeth, showering, or even putting my clothes on would exhaust all the air in my lungs and was cause to hurriedly reach for the oxygen mask.

Three or four months prior to transplant, I had to consider whether or not continuing to go to work was a smart thing to do, or even possible any longer. I was so physically weakened and vulnerable by then that any contagious bacteria, whether airborne or otherwise, was a serious danger to me. Again, I manage a restaurant, where money—we all know what germs money carries, handshakes, and unblocked sneezes and coughs—are constantly exchanged.

I brought my oxygen tank to work once, with the intent of going into the bathroom or a private area, use it as needed, and return to the floor, fresh as a daisy. This was not successful. After all, a manager walking around a restaurant with a plastic tube protruding from his nostrils is not the best look for enhancing other's appetites, believe it or not. So for the first time in forty years, twenty-two of them in this restaurant, I physically could not go to work at all.

So it was that when I did go out to walk my dog, go shopping, or the like, I would be carrying an oxygen tank slung over my shoulder with the plastic tube connected to it protruding from my nose.

Often, as many times as we might repeat our chosen mantras, it is not always to a successful end.

Clamshells

People awaiting lung transplants are often doing so for many months or even years. Many of these people are in dire straits and dependent on oxygen around the clock while waiting for their call. I recently met a gentleman, a fellow CFer, who underwent a bilateral lung transplant a little over one year ago. He is one of three brothers, the middle brother actually, who were all unfortunate enough to be born with this disease. There were no other children in the family. Three boys, all three with CF, not only goes against the percentages but is also extremely unfortunate for the whole family, certainly emotionally and possibly financially as well.

He is forty-one years old now and doing relatively well. After talking with him for a while, I realized how fortunate I was regarding the short amount of time I had to wait for my new lungs. Where I needed oxygen for only a few months prior to my surgery, this gentleman was basically bedridden for over a year, with constant oxygen flowing. Where my lungs were functioning at only 19 percent of capacity, a very low number, his lungs were working at only 6 percent of capacity.

I remember all too vividly when my lungs were at their weakest. With any activity, even with a strong flow of oxygen, I struggled mightily to get a breath. It's hard even for me to imagine the sense of suffocation he must have experienced with only 6 percent of his lungs working. With perhaps only days left before he would succumb, he received his transplant. As far as the status of his two brothers, the older is in his late forties and doing relatively well and the younger, in his thirties, is now awaiting transplant. Hopefully, all three will win their personal battles against our disease. Indeed, they may already have.

Lung transplantation was first attempted, with little to no success in 1963. Just the fact that they were "experimenting" with these surgeries was a monumental step for people with CF and various other lung diseases. In the earliest stages, only single lung transplants were being attempted. With transplant surgical procedures and rejection medications in their respective infancies, progress was extremely slow, which I am sure was to be expected.

Years passed and with continued research, medical trials, and the perseverance of a handful of doctors and scientists, by the mid-1970s, lung transplants were taking place. A rejection medication called cyclosporine was used at this time but was not overwhelmingly successful. Life expectancy post transplant was still only in the range of hours to days. With the lack of proven, successful rejection meds, the patients that made it through the surgery, and most did, had no real positive quality of life to speak of.

Continued suffering, though perhaps a different form of suffering post transplant, was in store for these desperate patients. It was for this reason, that when my sister Valerie was offered the chance to travel to Texas for bilateral lung transplantation in 1976, she heeded Dr. Gorvoy's advice and declined. She had tuberculosis by that juncture in her life, and this, combined with end stage CF, completely exhausted any energy she might have had in reserve at that point. Most of these transplant surgeries were single lung and because both lungs in the CF person are affected, both would have to be removed. These factors, and the difficult travel that would have been required, dictated their decision on this matter.

It wasn't until 1988 that the first CF patient underwent a "successful" bilateral lung transplant. This patient was able to survive only a few days, post transplant. It was a huge step forward though as both lungs were transplanted successfully in a CF patient for the first time.

Again, the immunosuppressants or rejection drugs in use at the time were still being experimented with, and progress along those lines continued to be extremely slow going. Since the surgical procedure itself has vastly improved over time, the success of these rejection medications remains the biggest obstacle regarding improvement in quality of life and life expectancy for all transplant recipients—lungs, kidney, heart and any other.

Early lung transplantation, from what I've learned through research, must have been extremely difficult not only for the patient but the doctor as well. Before the transplant could be performed, the patient's sternum, along with a few of the ribs, had to be cracked or cut so the surgeon could gain access to the chest cavity and perform the operation.

The new lungs were actually slipped under the ribs and sternum and all necessary *connections* were then lined up and sewn into place. Having gone through the post surgery pain that I experienced, with no broken bones, I can only imagine the pain that the earlier transplant patients endured. There are, even today, circumstances during lung transplants that dictate the sternum be broken so access to the lungs can be attained.

The transplant surgery I was to undergo is called a "clamshell" operation. It may sound a little crude, but it is truly called this, and for obvious reasons as I'll explain. With this procedure, one long incision is made, starting from below one armpit, across the length of the chest, under the breasts and ending under the opposite armpit. The chest is then lifted up along this incision, just like a clamshell. The surgeon is able, more simply, to perform the extraction of the old lungs and the insertion of the new while the "shell" is kept open. No broken bones...amazing.

Thank you to all those patients that volunteered to undergo lung transplants in those early years, when they knew the chance of survival was slim and the quality of their life would probably be poor. Your incredible bravery and the sacrifices you made so that those of us to follow might live a better life is appreciated beyond words.

Happy Fiftieth

To live fifty years with a tough strain of cystic fibrosis is a difficult task that will someday, hopefully soon, be the median age for all stricken with the disease. For my generation of CFers, fifty years of life has been very difficult to reach and an awful lot to ask.

Remembering that in the fifties and early sixties, for a CF born child, a year or so of life, if that, were to be expected. The milder the strain of CF, the better the chance of a longer life he or she will have, of course. To reiterate, I do not fall into the "mild" category, sad to say. That was why for me to reach that half century milestone was quite a big deal for me and all those who love me and know my struggle with the disease.

I recall joking with friends while in high school about not worrying too much about how much I drank or beat up my body. I would just say it didn't really matter; I probably wouldn't be here that long. When I think of those times, it reminds me of what Mickey Mantle, my childhood baseball idol, said in his last interview before he passed. I cannot quote him word for word, but suffice to say if he knew he was going to live as long as he did, he would have taken better care of himself. Of course, looking back, I wish I did.

My wife threw me a wonderful fiftieth birthday party with friends and family. This was a very special and emotional day for me, to say the least. To have my whole family, close relatives, my great friends, and Dr. Gorvoy and his amazing wife, Florence, with me to celebrate will be a memory I will look back on fondly.

My niece, Alana, read a beautiful letter to me written by her and Lara that I will cherish for as long as I live. The words in that letter and the words of congratulations on reaching the fifty-year milestone from all my loved ones are forever tattooed on my heart.

The Call of Life

Shortly after my celebration of the big *five*-o, I was listed, activated and now waiting for "the call" from Columbia Presbyterian Hospital. This would be the call telling me my new lungs are on their way.

MaryAnne had been witnessing firsthand the frustrating struggle I had been going through just to get through each day. She knew my lungs were working at only 19 percent capacity and failing but still was nervous about me undergoing the surgery. She had known me for thirty-three years at this point and has seen all the luck I've had with illness and certain medical procedures during that span. Not much of that luck, good. However, Dr. Sonnet, chief of thoracic surgery at Columbia, sat her down and explained that without the transplant, I wouldn't see another Christmas. This quickly did the trick as she realized this wasn't elective surgery, and we moved forward.

Having gone through all the medical and psychological exams, coordination of insurance companies and whatever else the preparation for transplant entailed, I was now ready to play the waiting game.

This is the only part of this whole transplant ordeal that worried me, the waiting. My blood type is B negative, not a common blood type, unfortunately, and those with rare blood types can wait months if not years for their organs, lungs, or otherwise. So I wasn't real confident that I would be called any time soon. Of course, not only blood type matches between the donor and recipient are necessary before you can proceed with the surgery. The donor must also match organ size, tissue, and the organ must be of good quality before the doctors will okay them for the recipient.

To this day, and to my last day on Earth, I will always be amazed and thankful that in spite of all I had going against me in early 2007, after only six to seven weeks on the list, I was called to Columbia Presbyterian Hospital. I was told there were lungs on the way to the hospital for me. I was excited of course!

My wife and I had gone through the steps we would follow when the call came. We made the necessary calls to our family and friends. The only thing that made me sad about leaving the house was leaving my four-legged friend, Sheena, for a couple of weeks. Now, as long as we didn't get a flat during the forty-five minute ride in, we'd be good to go.

I'm not going to bore you with all the details of getting prepped for surgery. Suffice to say I was all wired up to the massive heart and lung machine, IVs in a number of places, numerous doctors and nurses all in place and ready to go.

I loved watching it. This was better than the show, ER could ever be. This is a live performance of the highest order, with the characters all ready to play their part. I have always loved watching medical staffs in action, perhaps because I have lived my whole life around it. I am impressed by the professionalism and precision displayed by all involved. Back in 1987, while I was lying on the gurney, prior to my pancreas surgery, despite the pain I was in, I remember being amazed at the way everyone was preparing to go to work. All those in the operating room had a job to do and they all went about their important roles effortlessly, yet meticulously.

So here I am, in the operating room, hooked up and ready for transplant. Family and friends have been already been in the waiting room for a few hours now. The door to the OR opens, Dr. Davidio, the thoracic surgeon on call, pops his head in, shakes it east and west, and so ended my first attempt and "dry run" at transplant.

One of the tests the surgeon performs on the donor lungs before they can be transplanted is simply to fill the lungs with oxygen. Healthy lungs will retain or hold that oxygen for a few moments before deflating. These lungs did not, and deflated immediately.

My only request after the first "no go" attempt was for the medical team to hold off on starting an arterial line, or IV. This thickly gauged needle is inserted into the artery of one of the patient's wrists just as with a blood gas. This can be somewhat painful in spite of the numbing agent they may use on the area prior to insertion. After being told on my first attempt at transplant the donor lungs failed to stay inflated, the subsequent removal of this arterial line took place and was very painful. You would think the removal would be a relief, but extreme pressure must be put on the sight of the insertion so the blood clots as quickly as possible. I whined just enough about holding off on this aspect of surgical preparation, and for future attempts at transplant my wish would be granted.

Again, to my amazement, only three weeks later, another individual with a B negative blood type and matching lung size and tissue had died. This was a kind of luck I've never experienced and so soon after the first call.

On this occasion, chief thoracic surgeon, Dr. Sonnett, again found these lungs unsuitable for transplant. He informed me, while I was still on the operating table that had I been in absolute desperate condition at that time, he would have gone on with the surgery. The donor's lungs were not in great condition, and I believe he also was a smoker, which never helps. The surgeon wants, of course, to always transplant the strongest, healthiest lungs possible so that the recipient of those organs is given the best chance at survival and longevity. I, of course, agreed fully with Dr. Sonnett's decision.

I returned home once again but not quite as disappointed with this negative outcome as I was with the first failed attempt. The fact is that only fifty percent of lungs that are "harvested," as doctors put it, are healthy enough for transplant. Sometimes, the lungs will look great, Dr. Sonnett told me, but for whatever reason they don't pass certain criteria required for surgery.

I did some research prior to my transplant about certain procedures used to test the lungs but had absolutely no idea that only half the lungs that become available to the recipients are good enough for transplantation. I found that bit of information fascinating and a little depressing. I just always assumed, as far back as high school, when I knew I would someday need new lungs, that once you got called, that was it, you got your new lungs.

After this second try at transplant, I did become a bit frustrated and a little nervous that it could now be a long time before I would get another opportunity. I needed to hang on a while longer. The odds just can't be good for another unfortunate individual with a B negative blood type and my size to pass away. What a thing to hope for.

Maybe you can begin to understand the gamut of emotions one goes through while waiting for and then receiving someone else's organs to help you prolong your life. It's one of those situations that are hard to comprehend unless you've gone through it. I sincerely hope none of my readers have to know that unsettling feeling.

Believe it or not, only about four weeks later I received a third call from Columbia telling me to get over to the hospital as soon as I could. By now, I was programmed to expect a negative outcome regarding this new pair of lungs.

Still nervous and excited though, I once again was traveling on the Cross Bronx Expressway toward what I hoped would be my hospital for many years to come. It wasn't long before all the necessary wires and tubes again were in place.

Dr. Davidio opened the OR door, shook his head north and south and smiled at me. My heart raced, I smiled, and was ready to go.

From start to finish, or from admission to discharge, though it seemed like about a month, only ten days passed. This is exactly the time frame doctors want their transplant patients to adhere to, if possible. Understandably, they want you out of the hospital as soon as possible. Most people know that despite being a health care facility, within its walls, a constant bombardment of germs and bacteria, airborne, and otherwise, are taking place. With a transplant patient's compromised immune system, this is the worst place to be. This especially holds true for lung transplant patients. Unlike transplanting kidneys, hearts, livers, and body concealed organs, the lungs are constantly being exposed, with every breath, to all particles in the air around them.

Thank you Dr. Davidio and Dr. Sonnett for making the decisions you both did to wait a bit longer for these "healthy" lungs. I'm still here because of your discretions *and* your wonderful hands.

Vertigo

Opening my eyes for the first time in the ICU, though still a bit blurry, remains a vivid memory I'm sure I will carry with me always. Since I had been through major surgery before, I thought I knew what to expect. However, where there had been two chest tubes protruding from my body following the pancreas surgery, there were now four. The respirator tube was still down my throat, and I'm sure, after awakening, five minutes didn't pass before I asked for that uncomfortable thing to be removed. "Let's go...take this thing out, and let's try these new lungs out!" The nurses did take the respirator tube out shortly after my requests, or my pestering, whichever you prefer.

All my vital signs were taken and were stable. That was a relief, but I wouldn't be going anywhere for a couple of days. With some anesthesia and pain medication still "on board," as the doctors put it, I was uncomfortable but not in any real pain at that point. I was breathing comfortably, which was the one thing I noticed right away after the breathing tube was removed, but as the hours passed, that became the only thing that remained comfortable.

As the pain meds began to wear off, the reality of what my body had been through soon became evident. I wasn't able to move much as I lay in bed due to the chest tubes, a tube attached in my lower region we don't want to talk or think about, and the circus of wires and IVs that encompassed me. There was one more reason I couldn't and actually didn't want to move around too much while in the ICU.

I seriously feel for people who have now or have had problems in the past with vertigo. I know some of those who have had to deal with some mild vertigo, one of them being my mother. It is not a condition that is life-threatening, but it can be a condition that is life-altering.

Two months prior to my transplant, I was hospitalized in LIJH for a pneumonia infection. Due to my weakness and susceptibility to further complications from bacteria in the hospital, I was isolated in a special unit. While there, I was given the medication, Tobramycin, intravenously.

The antibiotic chosen for someone with infection is determined by which medication is "sensitive" to, or has the best chance of working against that particular germ or organism. Many of these medications, though helpful in clearing up an infection, can have adverse side effects, some of which can be severe, to those given them.

I had been on Tobra many times before in my life, with no side effects or complications. This time though, perhaps due to a higher dosage of the medicine than in the past, or just some bad luck, I developed vertigo as a result. I clearly recall the moment the vertigo set in.

I awoke one morning during that stay in LIJ, sat up, and felt a little dizzy and tipsy as though I had a few cocktails. I actually giggled at the feeling for a moment as it took my mind off the fact that I was in the hospital once again with pneumonia. This tipsy feeling amused me for about twenty minutes. It then became less amusing as the minutes and then the hours passed. This was, as I came to find out later that afternoon, "full blown" vertigo, my term for it.

Doctors told me there is no actual cure for this condition. There are some medications that can be taken to ease the nausea that accompanies vertigo, but after that, you're on your own.

Vertigo is caused by damage to the inner ear, in my case, that damage was caused by a reaction to the antibiotic running through my bloodstream. The condition can last a couple of days, weeks, months or for the rest of your life. The doctors have no idea how long each case they come across will last. This was bad news for me, especially before transplant, because I knew I had to stay active and strong immediately after the transplant. Having to hold on to nurses, railings, and my wife, post transplant will just not work for me.

So when the call came for my third try at transplant, here I was, going into the surgery with acute vertigo. A pattern of the luck I've experienced in my life has now emerged...would you agree? When I awoke after the surgery, of course I still had vertigo. Physical rehabilitation will not go as smoothly or as quickly as I had hoped it would.

Of course, the surgeons and pulmonologists want their transplant patients up and around the same day they are brought from the intensive care unit to their room. I did get up that first day but not without some help from my nurse and a walker. The trauma and weakness one experiences as a result of transplant surgery can be severe, but with vertigo added to the mix, rehab for me was definitely going to be behind schedule. I have a lot of luck, most of it not good. I will now apologize to my sister, Valerie for the self-pity I'm now displaying.

Dr. Davidio, my transplant surgeon, came up to see me the first day I was transferred to my own room. Upon witnessing me struggling with my balance while holding a walker and leaning on a nurse, he commented "You're making me look bad, Richie." The doctor was only half joking, but they do want their patients up and around, looking healthy and strong as quickly as humanly possible. The nurse then enlightened him regarding my physically unbalanced status. "That is a shame about the vertigo, but I still want Richie up four to five times a day," he responded swiftly and firmly.

The vertigo lasted two more months, bringing the total to four, before it lessened and over the course of a few days disappeared. The aggravating part of this whole issue is that with a compromised immune system, I will incur infections from time to time, whether sinus or lungs, and there will be times that Tobramycin will be the only antibiotic that has a chance to remedy that problem.

When infection does happen, vertigo will always take a back seat to possible spread of that infection and possible rejection. Give me all the Tobramycin I need, Doc. This four month episode was difficult and frustrating, but now is not the time to "throw in the white towel." There are rounds and battles yet to fight.

The Patch

There would be one or two more unpleasant hurdles I would have to clear before my discharge from Columbia.

About twelve years prior to my transplant, I was put on a Duragesic patch prescribed by my neurologist. The patch itself, which contained the narcotic, Fentanyl, looks like any nicotine patch you have seen, and as with a nicotine patch, the medicine is slowly released into your bloodstream through the pores in your skin. Fentanyl is one of the narcotics anesthesiologists use to put patients to sleep prior to surgery or other procedures requiring the patients to be unconscious. The reason I was started on this patch was to help keep the intermittent pain I was still experiencing from pancreatitis to a minimum. This wasn't a strong dosage of Fentanyl, but over time, this medication reached a level in my system whereby I rarely had to deal with any severe stomach pain.

I explained the reason for the patch to Dr. Davidio and requested he remove the patch during the transplant surgery as I knew I would be on a morphine drip for a couple of days post surgery. I hated that patch for many years and had wanted to come off it a number of times. This seemed like the perfect opportunity to do so. The doctors agreed, and it was removed in the operating room.

I knew that eventually, when the morphine drip dosage was reduced then discontinued, there would be a major price to pay in the form of withdrawals. Those who have been addicted to a narcotic, alcohol, or certain other mind altering drugs, you are familiar with the physical and psychological torture, and I don't use that word loosely, that your body and mind must go through when the drug is no longer introduced to your bloodstream.

To give you an idea of what the forty-eight hours immediately following the discontinuation of the morphine was like, let's just say hell would have been a few steps if not a few floors up. I've actually thought of sending Stephen King descriptions of some of the nightmares and "daymares" I went through during those withdrawals. Bizarre, gruesome, and horrifying describe them pretty well. However, I'm still here, so I obviously managed to get through it all by the time I was discharged.

Those ten days, between the vertigo and the withdrawals, oh yeah, and a double lung transplant, were some of the hardest rounds of fighting I will ever know and will never forget.

Broncho Buster

Follow up appointments post transplant are frequent, especially for the first six months after discharge. All transplant patients are closely monitored for any signs of rejection as those first few months post surgery are crucial. Patients are at their most vulnerable to infection at this juncture.

A number of bronchoscopies will be performed during these months looking for any signs of rejection. A bronchoscopy is a procedure whereby the doctor feeds a long thin scope down through the nose and throat to look directly into the lungs. A very small piece of the lung is cut out for biopsy, again, looking for rejection signs.

Bronchs, as the doctors call them, are also done to clear the lungs of any mucus buildup that may have accumulated in the lungs and airways as a result of the tremendous amount of anesthesia given for this lengthy surgical procedure. So begins the last dramatic, traumatic, and life-threatening event I will share with you, I promise.

Two to three days after arriving home from Columbia, I began to feel a slight rumbling in my throat and airways. Of course, I knew what it was immediately.

The rumbling was the thick mucus in my chest, leftover from the surgery beginning to break up. This mucus is a much thicker and pastier consistency than what had been "normal" for me. When it does start to break up it is difficult, to almost impossible, to cough out. The process of clearing this crap out is made more difficult due to the intense pain with each cough I experienced as a result of my chest wide incision.

After a day or two, I was becoming very frustrated with this rumbling in my airways, a discomfort I thought I was finished with, so I held my chest and forced a strong cough out. With that, some of this gluey substance broke loose, traveled up my airways and lodged itself at the base of my throat. "That was a good move, Rich, now I can't breathe at all." I remember telling myself

MaryAnne was sitting by me at the time and did not realize at first what was happening. I gestured to her that I could not breathe, but what could she do? As I sat, tears in my eyes and in a slight panic, as I was suffocating, I was finally, after what seemed like five minutes, able to create a pinhole in the mucus with a strong inhale. I continued to gasp for breath through this small hole until the hole eventually widened and my breathing was slowly eased.

I was so terrified of this happening again, and I knew it would, that I called a friend of ours, a nurse from Winthrop Hospital here on Long Island.

Colleen, who primarily assists in brain surgeries as an operating room nurse, is one of the strongest-minded, bravest, and caring people I will ever know.

I was confident and calm when she promptly arrived at my home. I was purposely breathing slowly and as calmly as I could so I wouldn't disturb or loosen any further the crap lining my airways. I brought Colleen up to my den, sat down, and it wasn't long before a cough ensued. The result of this cough was the same as had been earlier as I knew it would be. Although Colleen was sitting right next to me, I again began to panic as I struggled to create another pinhole to breathe through. Colleen kept me as calm as she could, rubbing my back and reassuring me I would break through and breathe again. Eventually, as you might have guessed, I did create another hole, but it was now clear that another trip to Columbia would be called for immediately.

As scary and nerve-racking as the forty-five minute ride to the hospital would be, there was no choice here. During the ride, I once again maintained a very slow cadence with my breathing. I allowed myself once or twice, a gentle clearing of my throat, praying to the God of Throats while I did so. Thankfully, I arrived at Columbia's emergency room with no further incidents.

The emergency room was as crowded as ever, even at twelve-thirty in the morning. I was put into one of the many depressing little rooms that lined the full perimeter of this hectic room. I'm not sure and who's counting but this may have been the 175th or 176th time I have been in an ER, so I am very familiar with the nurses and doctor's protocol.

I knew that it would undoubtedly be hours before a doctor will see me. Normally, this wouldn't bother me, but due to the terrifying hours prior, I became more agitated about the length of time I would most likely have to wait.

At two-thirty, I sent MaryAnne home, knowing I was going to be here for the long haul. I needed a bronchoscopy, and it was now a matter of when I would be able to get this procedure done.

I called a nurse into my room at about three o'clock and told her the rumbling in my chest and throat was getting worse. After informing me the doctors were all busy, as I had already brilliantly deduced, she left the room and returned with some sort of plastic pump, with a two-foot plastic tube attached. Can you guess what this device is?

"If you start to choke, put some petroleum jelly on this end, stick it down your throat and begin pumping manually," she said. Really? So now I'm qualified, with zero medical training, to be performing an invasive, dangerous procedure while, by the way, I'm suffocating. I'll most likely be panicking, but I'll gently feed this tube down my throat and begin to pump this vile crap out of me? As interesting and pleasurable as that sounds, I don't think so. I believe I would rather have the professional give it a try, thank you.

I finally relaxed enough to actually lay back on the gurney and get a little rest. About five in the morning, with no warning, an involuntary cough came out of nowhere, and my worst fear became reality.

I ran, and I mean ran out of the room up to the desk in the ER and started banging my fists to get the nurses' and doctors' attention. Loud noises *do* attract attention, so this method alerted them to the fact that I could not breathe. By now, at least a minute had passed since the mucus became lodged in my throat, and by the time a doctor came to my aid, I was in full panic mode.

He sat me down and did basically the same thing Colleen did and tried to keep me as calm as possible until, once again, I created a small hole to breathe through. Why didn't the doctor put that tube down my throat? Was it because he hadn't had the same extensive training in the procedure as I had?

Anyway, with tears running down my cheeks, snot running down my nose, shaking and exhausted, I was once again breathing relatively calmer but thinking that the bronchoscopy couldn't come fast enough.

Two hours later, my doctor performed the procedure, and I was sent home clean as a whistle with no further complications. This was a tough and scary round of boxing to get through, but I cannot and will not fail in my quest to beat this goddamn disease back.

Feeling a bit Squamous

I will always be the first to admit that as I was growing up, I definitely was a bit preoccupied with my looks. One might even say I had a problem with vanity. I believe I've mentioned this already. Because of this, I thank the heavens that what happened to my beautiful face three years ago, didn't happen while I was a much younger man. Of course, I will explain this...one of the oddest thing to ever happen to me in my crazy life.

Those of us with little or no immune system are constantly at risk for all manner of health problems. Most of you are probably aware of this fact. One of the more difficult and sometimes dangerous issues our compromised immune systems have to deal with is numerous forms of skin cancer.

I was told by my doctors that more than likely I would have to deal with some form of skin cancer. The three basic types of skin cancer are basal, the least harmful; squamous, which if not detected early, can spread quickly to the lymph nodes, possibly becoming life-threatening; and melanoma, which is the least "preferred" cancer and is life-threatening if not identified in its early stages.

Let me preface what occurred in my case by first stating that one of the few advantages, shall we say, of being on antibiotics since infancy is that I have never had to deal with acne. I knew this fact as a young teenager, and after seeing what some of my friends had to go through, believe me, I was grateful for that. Once in a while, a zit or two would pop up, but I never had to deal with multiple acne eruptions.

So how many of you have ever gotten a pimple on your lip? Please raise your hands. Those who have, certainly know how painful that can be and to get rid of.

In 2009, when I spotted the beginning of a tiny pimple on my upper lip, I didn't think much of it only to realize I would have to wait a few days to, excuse me, pop it. That's right, zit popping; I enjoy keeping my readers riveted with such stories. Wait, it does get better.

A few days passed and this little pimple grew a bit in size, but I was still unable to get rid of it. Sensing it wasn't a normal pimple (as opposed to an abnormal pimple), I made an appointment to see my dermatologist, but of course I had to wait a week for an appointment. In that span of time, the growth of this entity became somewhat aggressive. The size of a very large zit now, I became really frustrated with it. I proceeded to go into the bathroom and pinch it as hard as I could without passing out. This was so painful, tears were pouring out, and not from crying. Blood, and a lot of it, was the only thing that came out as a result. After a minute or so, I stopped.

When I finally met with the dermatologist, he prescribed an ointment to take care of it. As it turned out, this was a huge misdiagnosis. In retrospect, I should have asked why he wasn't taking a piece of it to biopsy, knowing my immune system was compromised. Live and learn because I will always speak up from here on in about anything I have concerns about regarding my health, and otherwise. The doctor, had he moved on this quickly, would have saved me a lot of anguish and pain…and lip. This pimple was eventually diagnosed as an aggressive form of squamous cell skin cancer.

I tried desperately to get an appointment with a new dermatologist recommended to me by a friend. My new and improved dermatologist proceeded to biopsy this little monster, now about the size of a dime, and another week passed before I was told the result. I then had to coordinate appointments with both an oncology and plastic surgeon to have it removed. The procedure would take place at my old hospital, North Shore LIJ, but would take another two weeks before we could have both surgeons available.

By the time I was able to have the surgery, this growth on my upper lip was applying for its own zip code and was the size of a quarter. This was, by far and away, the freakiest thing, and I'm talking medical journal material that I'd ever seen, and it has now made itself a home, zip code, and all on my lip.

The surgery was performed and about 40 percent of the tissue my upper lip was comprised of taken out to ensure that all the cancer had been removed. This round of fighting was mercifully over and I am now slightly less handsome than I was before.

Paying it Forward

I have recently written a second letter of thanks and appreciation to the family whose loved one's lungs are keeping me alive. I will continue to do so every five years from the day of my transplant just to let them know how I am doing. So I should have about another four or five letters to write. Now *that's* a confident attitude, or is that arrogant, I'm not sure.

The gift I have received from my organ donor can never be repaid, but I can at least continue to show my "undying," pardon the pun, gratitude. It certainly must be a difficult and emotional decision for them to contact, let alone meet in person, the individual whose body houses their loved one's organs. I can only speak to the emotions I know I would go through by meeting the family face–to-face.

The donor family has yet to respond to my letters and that's okay. I would, as hard as I'm sure it would be for me, love to be able to stand in front of them and show them how well I'm doing. If this meeting ever takes place, I will promise them that I will do my best to stay strong and to pay their loved one's generosity forward in all the ways I am able.

I had never heard the phrase *pay it forward* until a number of years ago when the movie of the same name was released. I love the phrase and moreover, the concept. Do wish I had coined the phrase myself.

When I initially considered committing my time and effort to writing this memoir, one of the subjects I wanted to touch on were the people, young and old, either born with CF or parents of a CF child, I have spoken to about my life with this disease.

As a young teen, I recall one of my hospitalizations when a young parent, after witnessing me rolling up and down the halls atop the base of the IV pole, asked if she could speak with me when I was finished with my "busy" schedule. The woman had a son only a couple of years younger than I, also with CF, and not doing too well. She, of course, did not know what the future held for her son.

The young mother was not only surprised but encouraged that despite the IV tubes sticking out of my arms and the knowledge that I also had CF (she must have asked the nurses), I still had the strength and energy to do what I was doing. Looking back, perhaps my first words of advice to her should have been to see if her son somehow could acquire a good case of OCD. That would have been a good start.

We spoke for a while and she then asked if I would talk to her son about his future with cystic fibrosis. I introduced myself to the boy, and we spoke for about an hour, or should I say, I spoke for about an hour. Though he was discouraged with the way he was feeling at the time, I persuaded him to get up and move around as opposed to lying in bed and sulking. I think the fact that we were so close in age almost embarrassed him into taking some action to improve and strengthen himself.

With cystic fibrosis, if you stay active, you can live a happy life, no matter how long it may be. If, on the other hand, you stay physically stagnant, you will soon be depressed, become lazy, and live miserably until you no longer are. I've been there, and he knew it. For someone else, including his mother, father, or even his doctor, to tell him the same, will not and cannot have the same impact. Talking to the boy for a while had a calming effect on him and his mother, I'm sure.

I knew, even as a young man, how emotionally difficult and frustrating it is for any child with CF. I really didn't know the reason why, but I've always felt compelled to talk to and do what I can to ease the anguish these children, teens, and their parents go through with this disease. As I've mentioned before, I have always offered, and have taken part in clinical trials and various other tests associated with advancing the search for improved medications, therapies, and of course, a cure for cystic fibrosis.

I continue to pay it forward in these ways where and whenever I can. The effort put forth on my behalf by not only Dr. Gorvoy but all the many doctors, nurses, and technicians that kept me alive as an infant, then as a young boy and now as an adult, has been extraordinary.

I had always felt and still feel an overwhelming sense of responsibility to make the result of their efforts something they can be proud of. To keep a child born of a disease with no cure and with almost no chance of survival alive all these years is not just extraordinary but miraculous in my opinion.

I owe thanks to too many people to even try and count for helping me fight through all those infections and diseases. Now, due to my successful transplant, I have new reasons to be thankful and to assume the responsibility of helping in any way I can, pre transplant and post transplant CF patients. I am strongly compelled to continue to *pay it forward.*

Amazing Things

"Amazing things are happening here" is the phrase that New York's Columbian Presbyterian Hospital uses as its credo. There truly *are* amazing things happening not only in New York's hospitals but hospitals and laboratories throughout the country and the world. In my lifetime alone, as far as CF is concerned, I have seen and benefitted from tremendous advancements in antibiotic therapies, physical therapies, and gene recognition through laboratory testing.

Indeed, in the relatively short "lifetime" of CF (1938) when compared to some other terminal diseases, we have seen significant strides in many areas. Transplant procedures, as I've mentioned, have improved with great speed in just the last ten years. In the last five years alone, one of the rejection drugs I had been originally prescribed has been replaced by an even more effective one with fewer side effects.

Life expectancy in CF patients and lung transplant patients continue to rise. I recently visited with my friend, Dr. Gorvoy, who has just turned ninety-four. His mind still astoundingly sharp as a tack; he recalls back in the fifties and sixties when the majority of CF children were not coming close to reaching adolescence.

As a matter of fact, he reminds me that it wasn't that long ago, relatively speaking, that CF was regarded and labeled as a childhood disease.

He allows himself now, when he rarely did before, to get a bit emotional as he remembers many of the children, including Valerie, who, even with the best medications of the time, he could not save from their suffering and eventual succumbing to the disease. His kind heart and unwavering compassion for these children and young adults, I can assure you, eased their suffering in a way only they could know. This compassion and love rained over them by this special man; let them pass in peace.

Of course, in spite of all advancements made in the field of pulmonary diseases, infants as well as adults stricken with CF still are at constant risk of the next deadly infection. To say there is still much work to be done before we can achieve the goal of a cure is an enormous understatement.

Thank God there are scientists and doctors still devoting their time and knowledge to help get us there. I would love to see that happen in my lifetime, of course, but realistically, I will be happy if more and more *amazing* things continue to happen toward the goal of knocking out CF. What I would give to see my *crib gloves* deliver the final blow.

Thanks to You

If I were to try and list all the people whose thoughts, prayers, and actions are the reason I'm sitting here, figuring out how to wrap up my book, it would be a practice in futility. I'm old, and there's no way I could remember them all. Suffice to say that starting from my childhood best buddy, Steve, who remains a treasured friend, through Peter, my great friend and partner in crime, many friends along the way have inspired me to want to live and laugh.

I only hope they know that the incredible hilarity and sense of humor I have brought into their lives was my way of saying thank you for how they've each impacted mine. I close my eyes and see everyone, from Spunky, Termite, Clem, Boagie and Swede, to Barbara, Jody, Nancy, and JoAnn, smiling as I write this.

All of my aunts and uncles have always shown unconditional love and support for me, as have my cousins, in anything I have done. The love that my family and relatives show each other when they get together is real with a depth that can't be measured. I have always been grateful for that and have never taken it for granted. I have witnessed, as we all have, many families torn apart by one thing or another. My large tribe of relatives has been very fortunate to not have this be the case for us. Their prayers for me, and I know there have been hundreds throughout my life, have helped and encouraged me beyond expression.

From Dr. Miller to Dr. Gorvoy and now Dr. Arcasoy and his physician's assistant, Nelani, I once again express to my readers how exquisitely blessed I have been to have such caring physicians and nurses to accompany me on my journey. They all have my lifelong undying respect and gratitude. They have not only kept me physically strong but mentally strong as well. I see these doctors working long hours, never surrendering to the pressures they face and never losing their wonderful bedside manner, and I am in awe. How can I not fight this goddamn disease with all the strength I have when they fight beside me?

I continue to visit Dr. Gorvoy, and we still discuss, among other things, upgraded therapies and medications for CF, and amazingly, he is up on all the latest. At ninety-four, an avid *New York Times* reader, he still has a vocabulary that will make your jaw drop.

There is no gratitude I can express to Dr. Gorvoy that would be thanks enough for what he has done for me. To live and fight CF as hard and as long as I can, help when I am able to continue his work with all my soul, and to pray for all the children that were and are now too ill for even him to save, will be my way of saying thank you.

My brothers and sisters are compassionate, giving and loving people who are that way because of the way they were raised. We didn't grow up in a house of anger or prejudice, and this is evident in how we've lived our lives. And it is a testament to how all of *their* children, I'm confident, will live their lives.

Perhaps without realizing, each of my siblings, in their own way has taken on some of the best character traits of our mother. We were basically raised by only our mother, and this could not have been easy for my younger siblings or my mother. Not really having a father present was especially tough on my three younger brothers. For the boys to have only limited memories of their father, and some of those not pleasant, was an issue they each had to reconcile with.

Because of the way my mother conducted herself with her children with understanding and much patience, I am very proud to say, despite some serious problems along the way, all of my family is intact, respectful, and loving of one another.

This could not have been an easy route for my mother, especially when it came to her oldest son. From what I understand, he was quite a handful for ten or twenty years. Nancy Keane turns eighty this May, and I hope we are both here to celebrate her ninetieth. She is that special kind of person who makes those who meet and get to know her want to be better human beings. I hope I have made her as proud of me as I am of her.

My drive to keep living, to stay on top of my medications, to keep moving, and stay active are reinforced every morning I awaken. Just waking up each day and seeing my wife and friend, MaryAnne, I am reminded how incredibly lucky I was forty years ago when I first met her.

There really aren't many like her in the world. To know the heartache she has been through, watching helplessly sometimes, the many physical and emotional difficulties I have dealt with, pushes me to live and love her awhile longer. I truly hope the laughter and love I have given her since the day I met her all those years ago, now continued through our marriage, has in some way made the journey worthwhile for her. My life means so much more, indeed still *having* a life to speak of, means so much more, because of MaryAnne. Thank you again for saving my life.

Keep Fighting

On December twentieth of 1976, I rode with my mother over to Long Island Jewish Medical Center to see Valerie. I knew, for all intents and purposes, this would be the last time I would talk to her. All that day I was consumed with what I would say to her. I wanted her to smile. I wanted to make her laugh. That was easy for me to do; she was my friend and my greatest audience. I was not and to this day, am not comfortable visiting anyone in the hospital, especially those very ill, despite having been on the other end of that visit many times.

I went in the room by myself as Mom waited in the hall. Now with tuberculosis, pneumonia and completely exhausted, Valerie's lungs were filled with so much fluid, there was no longer room for air enough to even cough. The dinner tray was across her lap and the head of the bed was completely upright, so she was in the seated position. Leaning on the table with arms folded and head resting face down on the tray, she heard me come in. She knew it was me but could not lift her head to look.

When I said a soft hello as I entered the room, all she could do was to lift her index finger to acknowledge me. It was then that all my plans of conversation went out the window. I sat on the bed next to Valerie, facing her, as I had done many times before. But this time, I couldn't pick my head up and could only look down at the bed or the floor.

A couple of minutes, which seemed like hours, passed before I could get my mind focused on what I had to say. Looking back, I wish I had said something soothing or loving or even mildly humorous. I was useless, unfortunately. I had my hand on her leg and my head down the whole time, not having the emotional strength or fortitude to look at her.

I finally lifted my head up, and all I was able to muster after all this preparation and thought were the words, "I don't know what to say, Val." Her response would be muffled by the oxygen mask covering her face, but she turned her head and looked at me, and this girl who had suffered so long was so ill and riddled with fever, said, "You have to keep fighting!"

I will never take these crib gloves off, and I will *never* stop fighting, Valerie.

Afterword

I realize I probably have used all the necessary clichés about what it's like growing up with cystic fibrosis at some point in my memoirs; CF is not who I am…CF doesn't live through me, I live through CF…and so on. These clichés can be used as effective mantras for some. For myself, and I believe many other CF people, they are words that are not only appropriate but indeed help reinforce and strengthen our resolve. Remember this: having any disease, be it cystic fibrosis, cancer, or the like, does not define who you are. How you respond to having that disease does.

We all have our own respective battles in life. At the finish of some of those battles we are triumphant, and some, we are not. Those people with CF and other incurable, life-threatening diseases are engaged in battles that are foreign to those outside that circle. The fact is though to know there are people out there fighting for their lives everyday does not diminish the importance or severity of the personal battles and trials all people go through. Here is one more cliché… everything is relative. We all have to remain strong to persevere in this difficult though beautiful world.

My goal in writing this memoir is twofold. First, I need to let other CFers, young and old, know that although the problems they may be having seem never ending, they are not alone in their difficult struggles. Second, I want my book to enlighten those who read it to the fact that the cure for cystic fibrosis, which will be here, is not yet. There is more that needs to be done and the CF foundation still needs much help to make "sixty-five roses" just a beautiful bouquet of flowers.

The fact is the great fortune that I had been born in 1956 with a tough strain of cystic fibrosis and am still here in 2013 has not been lost on me. I have fully enjoyed my life despite CF. As far as I'm concerned, any years I've had on this earth after my first birthday have been gravy.

For me, to be able to enjoy what is now six years of a life without coughing or congestion is a gift that I am grateful for far beyond words. To have only pills to take, an occasional antibiotic inhalation or IV, and almost no coughing after fifty years of it, is truly euphoric to me. I desperately hope the donor family who's loved one saved my life will read this so they fully understand what their gesture has done for me.

The doctors and scientists who work tirelessly, those who dedicate their time and money to various CF charities around the world, but mostly the infants, children, and adults who have been born into this world with our shared disease deserve a cure. I know it's on the way.

Dr. Jack Gorvoy, who passed away two months prior to the completion of my book, will look down from Heaven and smile proudly when the cure arrives.

I now ask everyone to put on their boxing gloves as I have mine. The fight continues.